HIKES LIST

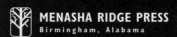
MENASHA RIDGE PRESS
Birmingham, Alabama

60 HIKES within 60 MILES

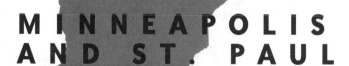

MINNEAPOLIS AND ST. PAUL

INCLUDING THE TWIN CITIES' GREATER METRO AREA AND BEYOND

THIRD EDITION

TOM WATSON

60 HIKES WITHIN 60 MILES: MINNEAPOLIS AND ST. PAUL

Copyright © 2012 Tom Watson
All rights reserved
Printed in the United States of America
Published by Menasha Ridge Press
Distributed by Publishers Group West
Third edition, second printing 2014

Library of Congress Cataloging-in-Publication Data

    Watson, Tom, 1947–
      60 hikes within 60 miles, Minneapolis and St. Paul : includes hikes
    in and around the Twin Cities / Tom Watson. — 3rd ed.
        p. cm. — (60 hikes within 60 miles)
    ISBN 978-0-89732-933-0 (pbk.) — ISBN 0-89732-933-3 ()
    1. Hiking—Minnesota—Minneapolis Metropolitan Area—Guidebooks.
    2. Hiking—Minnesota—Saint Paul Metropolitan Area—Guidebooks.
    3. Minneapolis Metropolitan Area (Minn.)—Guidebooks.
    4. Saint Paul Metropolitan Area (Minn.)—Guidebooks.
    I. Title. II. Title: Sixty hikes within sixty miles, Minneapolis and St. Paul.
    GV199.42.M62M569 2012
    796.5109776'579—dc23

                        2012012946 <tel:2012012946>

Cover and text design by Steveco International
Cover photo of Lake Calhoun, Minneapolis, Minnesota © YinYang
All interior photos by Tom Watson
Maps by Scott McGrew and Tom Watson

Menasha Ridge Press
P.O. Box 43673
Birmingham, AL 35243
menasharidge.com

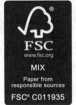 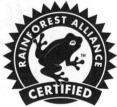

DISCLAIMER

TABLE OF CONTENTS

ACKNOWLEDGMENTS

IN THIS AGE OF ALMOST INSTANTANEOUS INFORMATION RETRIEVAL, I found that all the agencies in the Twin Cities that manage trails within their respective boundaries are very well wired when it comes to providing up-to-date information. The websites and contact numbers listed in the Appendix offer hikers a plethora of information on the trails and amenities of nearly every park in the Twin Cities.

The Three Rivers Park District has an incredible resource base of maps and information about each park in its domain.

The Minnesota Valley National Wildlife Refuge offers a daisy chain of park areas along the Minnesota River—one of the best scenic and wildlife viewing areas in the Twin Cities. Its information base, like its parks, continually improves with more helpful maps and brochures each year.

More useful descriptions of hiking areas and amenities are provided by the U.S. Fish & Wildlife Service. I don't believe there is one federal agency responsible for outdoor recreation that doesn't have useful information on hiking opportunities in its management areas.

On a more localized basis, each county and municipality has published maps and information charts highlighting which parks offer hiking trails. Armed with this information and a good map of the cities, one can literally hike from one end to the other, guided all the way with neighborhood information on trails and amenities.

The tourism departments of both Minnesota and Wisconsin feature hiking as a predominant recreation activity in their respective states. Each offers maps and general information as well as contact information for each recreational region of its state.

Minnesota's Department of Natural Resources (DNR), particularly the great people at the state park system, is yet another incredible source of information. A good number of the hikes in this book are found within state parks close to the Twin Cities, and information provided by the DNR enables a hiker to get a feel for the entire state just by sampling trails at these nearby areas.

Very special thanks to my sister, Lynn, whose invaluable research, ongoing hospitality, and support throughout this project will always be deeply appreciated.

FOREWORD

WELCOME TO MENASHA RIDGE PRESS'S *60 Hikes within 60 Miles,* a series designed to provide hikers with the information they need to find and hike the best trails surrounding cities usually underserved by guidebooks.

Our strategy was simple: First, find a hiker who knows the area and loves to hike. Second, ask that person to spend a year researching the most popular and best trails around. And third, have that person describe each trail in terms of difficulty, scenery, condition, elevation change, and other categories of information that are important to hikers. "Pretend you've just completed a hike and met up with other hikers at the trailhead," we told each author. "Imagine their questions, and be clear in your answers."

An experienced hiker and writer, author Tom Watson has selected 60 great hikes in and around the Twin Cities metropolitan area. From urban hikes that make use of parklands and streets to flora- and fauna-rich treks along the Mississippi to aerobic outings along the area's glaciated hills, Watson provides hikers (and walkers) with a wonderful variety of hikes— all within roughly 60 miles of Minneapolis and St. Paul.

You'll get more out of this book if you take a moment to read the Introduction, which explains how to read the trail listings. The "Topographic Maps" section will help you understand how useful topos will be on a hike and will tell you where to get them. And though this is a where-to rather than a how-to guide, those of you who have not hiked extensively will find the Introduction of particular value. As much for the opportunity to free the mind as to free the body, let these hikes elevate you above the urban hurry.

All the best,
The Editors at Menasha Ridge Press

ABOUT THE AUTHOR

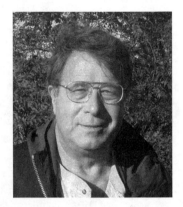

BORN IN CALIFORNIA, Tom Watson moved to the Twin Cities from Missouri at age 7. He remained in Minnesota until graduating from the College of Forestry of the University of Minnesota with a B.S. in Forest Resource Management/Recreation. Then, in the mid-1980s, Tom moved to Kodiak, Alaska, where he spent 15 years operating a sea-kayak touring business and began working as a freelance writer and photographer. Published in several national magazines and an active member of the Outdoor Writers Association of America and the Association of Great Lakes Outdoor Writers, Tom has won several awards for his articles. He is also the author of *Best Tent Camping Minnesota*. Besides hiking, his hobbies include photography, music, community theater, gardening, bird-watching, paddling, and camping.

PREFACE

SO MANY OPTIONS

WITHIN THE SEVEN-COUNTY METRO AREA that encompasses the Twin Cities of Minneapolis and St. Paul lies a network of hundreds of miles of trails. In the state of 10,000 lakes, nearly 1,000 of them lie within these urban borders. Consequently, Minneapolis has been dubbed the City of Lakes. Once you discover all the trails throughout this same area, you may be inclined to call the Twin Cities "The Cities of Trails."

Some of these trails are broad, paved corridors through multiuse parks generously developed to provide myriad recreational opportunities for the young and old, the robust trekker, and the casual stroller. Other trails are country lanes, walkways of grass winding through majestic stands of Minnesota hardwoods. Still others comprise a spiderweb network that might remind one of well-used deer trails.

Some are isolated within a pocket of greenery surrounded by vast ribbons of freeway concrete and broad subdivisions. Others are woven within the fabric of parklands so expansive that you could literally spend weeks hiking all the networks lying within their folds.

THE TRAILS INCLUDED

Wherever there was a network of trails, I tried to pick a trail that was representative of the area—one that showcased the park's or region's main attractions or personality. As you find certain areas more appealing, you will find other trails that you feel are equally exciting or challenging. That's the beauty of exploration and discovery. The trails cited in this guidebook are meant to introduce you to a particular hike and let your own wanderlust take it from there.

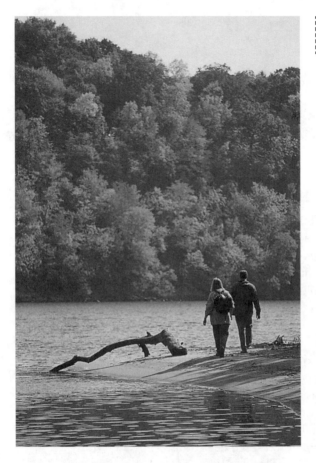

A couple walking along the
Mississipi River

I deliberately chose not to include the regional corridors that are part of this vast system of trails. These are wonderful pathways—the Luce Line trail that bisects the entire western region of the Twin Cities, the Hennepin Regional Trails, and the Scott County Regional Trail—many sections of which were reclaimed from discarded railroad rights-of-way. They are primarily bike corridors upon which you can also hike. They are great for connecting one park to another via greenbelts or low-traffic routes. I consider these the interstates and freeways of the hiking world. The trails covered in this book are more the back roads and neighborhood routes that really showcase the areas through which they pass.

A FEW CONSIDERATIONS

Most of the trail descriptions are self-explanatory. I am a moderate-paced hiker. I enjoy looking off the trail to the side as I go. I carry binoculars, as I am an avid birder.

I also bring along a camera and an appropriate lens combination for both scenic shots and close-ups of flowers and insects.

The maps have been produced from those available either at the park's visitor center or at a trailhead or kiosk information unit. Sometimes these maps don't offer quite as much information as you might need en route, particularly at intersections and path options. I've tried to fix most of those omissions. Common sense and a bit of dead reckoning should keep you well oriented. If you stay on the main trail, it's nearly impossible to become lost.

Some of the trails you'll encounter are multiuse (hiking and biking) trails by design. Sharing the route with cyclists means respecting their right-of-way as you would hope they respect yours. On some of the hikes, pedestrian and bike lanes are separated by subtle barriers or restraints; on others traffic is married onto the same pathway for the entire route. Be extra cautious at turns and hills; be courteous, and be safe.

Some of the trailheads for these hikes are heavily trafficked and others far less so, but theft is an unfortunate possibility at all of them. When you leave your car at a trailhead, park it well away from the road to reduce the likelihood of a collision, and be sure to lock it. Leave your valuables out of sight, and don't tempt thieves with open windows. The risks of theft and vandalism are minimal, but there's no reason not to take simple precautions that minimize them further.

GET OUT THERE

The descriptions in this guidebook profile trails ranging from a paved sidewalk around a neighborhood lake to former railroad grades to narrow paths along the

banks of the mighty Mississippi River. They were chosen to feature specific trails that best showcase the type and quality of natural or historical amenities within a park or area. Each hike opens the door to other possibilities within the same network of trails.

I encourage readers to use the information herein as a starting point to get to know a park or primitive area. Use this book like a menu: choose the hike that suits your tastes for a sample of the trail entrées each park has to offer. The portions are all within a day's range of hiking, and the bounty is quite fulfilling.

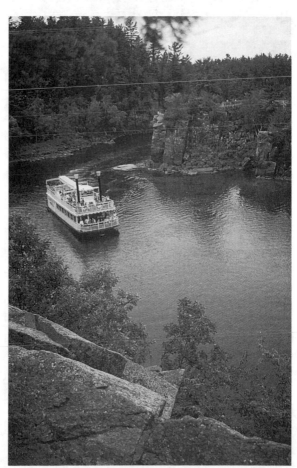

A paddlewheel boat on the
St. Croix River at Interstate Dells

RECOMMENDED HIKES

HIKE CATEGORIES

✓ 3 miles or less	✓ 5–10 miles	✓ flat terrain
✓ 3–5 miles	✓ >10 miles	✓ hilly terrain

▮ = easy ▮ = moderate ▮ = strenuous

REGION Hike #/Hike name	page	3 miles or less	3–5 miles	5–10 miles	> 10 miles	flat terrain	hilly terrain
URBAN-SUBURBAN ST. PAUL							
1 Battle Creek	18		▮				✓
2 Big Rivers Regional Trail	21		▮				
3 Crosby Farm Park	25	▮				✓	
4 Lake Elmo Park Reserve, Eagle Point Lake	29		▮			✓	
5 South St. Paul Riverfront Trail	33			▮		✓	
6 Thompson County Park, Thompson Trail	37	▮					
URBAN-SUBURBAN MINNEAPOLIS							
7 Bass Ponds Trail, Long Meadow Lake	42	▮				✓	
8 Bryant Lake	46	▮					
9 Bunker Hills Regional Park	49	▮					
10 Carlos Avery Trail	53			▮			
11 City Lakes Chain, Lakes Harriet, Calhoun, and Isles	57				▮	✓	
12 Clifton E. French Regional Park	61	▮					
13 Coon Rapids Dam	64	▮				✓	
14 Fort Snelling State Park, Snelling Lake and Pike Island Trails	67			▮		✓	
15 Hyland Lake Park Reserve, Richardson Interpretive Trail	70	▮					✓
16 Lake Nokomis	74	▮				✓	

REGION Hike #/Hike name	page	3 miles or less	3–5 miles	5–10 miles	> 10 miles	flat terrain	hilly terrain
URBAN-SUBURBAN MINNEAPOLIS *(continued)*							
17 Minnehaha Falls and Creek	78	ıll					✓
18 Mississippi Gorge Trail	82			ıll		✓	
19 Rice Creek North Regional Trail	87		ıll				✓
20 Wood Lake Nature Center	91	ıll				✓	
SOUTHWEST							
21 Cleary Lake Regional Park	98		ıll			✓	
22 Douglas State Trail	102			ıll			
23 Lake Byllesby Regional Park	105	ıll				✓	
24 Louisville Swamp, Mazomani Trail	108		ıll				
25 Minnesota Valley State Recreation Area, Lawrence Trail	113		ıll			✓	
26 Murphy-Hanrehan Park Reserve	117	ıll					✓
27 Sakatah Lake State Park	120	ıll					
SOUTHEAST							
28 Afton State Park	126		ıll				✓
29 Barn Bluff	130	ıll					✓
30 Cannon Valley Trail	134				ıll	✓	
31 Cottage Grove Ravine Regional Park	139	ıll					✓
32 Frontenac State Park, Bluffside Trail	142	ıll					✓
33 Lebanon Hills Regional Park, Holland/Jensen Lakes Loop	146	ıll					✓
34 Miesville Ravine Park Reserve	151		ıll				
35 Nerstrand–Big Woods State Park, Big Woods Trail	154		ıll				✓
36 Spring Lake Park Reserve, Schaar's Bluff Trail	158	ıll				✓	
NORTHWEST							
37 Baker Park Reserve	164			ıll			
38 Baylor Regional Park	168		ıll			✓	
39 Carver Park Reserve/Lowry Nature Center, Tamarack Trail	171	ıll				✓	
40 Crow-Hassan Park Reserve	175		ıll				

REGION Hike #/Hike name	page	3 miles or less	3–5 miles	5–10 miles	> 10 miles	flat terrain	hilly terrain
NORTHWEST *(continued)*							
41 Elm Creek Park Reserve	179				▪ıl	✓	
42 Elm Creek Park Reserve, Eastman Nature Trail	183		ıll				
43 Lake Maria State Park	188		ıll				✓
44 Lake Minnewashta Regional Park, Marsh Trail Loop	192	ıl					✓
45 Lake Rebecca Park Reserve	195			ıll		✓	
46 Rum River Central Regional Park	199	ıll				✓	
47 Rum River North County Park	203		ıll			✓	
48 Sand Dunes State Forest, Ann Lake	206	ıl					✓
49 Sherburne National Wildlife Refuge, Prairie's Edge Trail	209			ıll		✓	
50 Snail Lake	213		ıll			✓	
NORTHEAST							
51 Gateway State Trail	218			ıll			
52 Interstate State Park, Minnesota	222		ıll				
53 Interstate State Park, Wisconsin	226		ıll				✓
54 Kinnickinnic State Park, Wisconsin	231		ıll			✓	
55 Pine Point Regional Park Trail	234		ıll			✓	
56 Red Cedar State Trail, Wisconsin	238				ıll	✓	
57 Tamarack Nature Center	242	ıll				✓	
58 Wild River State Park	245		ıll				
59 William O'Brien State Park, Upper Park Trail	249		ıll				✓
60 Willow River State Park	253		ıll				✓

MORE RECOMMENDED HIKES

HIKE CATEGORIES

- ✓ multiuse trails
- ✓ kids
- ✓ flora
- ✓ bird-watching
- ✓ fall foliage
- ✓ historical sites
- ✓ geographical features

REGION Hike #/Hike name	page	multiuse trails	kids	flora	bird-watching	fall foliage	historical sites	geographical features
URBAN-SUBURBAN ST. PAUL								
1 Battle Creek	18	✓						
2 Big Rivers Regional Trail	21							
3 Crosby Farm Park	25					✓	✓	
4 Lake Elmo Park Reserve, Eagle Point Lake	29							
5 South St. Paul Riverfront Trail	33	✓						✓
6 Thompson County Park, Thompson Trail	37							
URBAN-SUBURBAN MINNEAPOLIS								
7 Bass Ponds Trail, Long Meadow Lake	42		✓		✓		✓	
8 Bryant Lake	46	✓						
9 Bunker Hills Regional Park	49	✓						
10 Carlos Avery Trail	53	✓						
11 City Lakes Chain, Lakes Harriet, Calhoun, and Isles	57							
12 Clifton E. French Regional Park	61							
13 Coon Rapids Dam	64	✓						
14 Fort Snelling State Park, Snelling Lake and Pike Island Trails	67	✓					✓	

REGION Hike #/Hike name	page	multiuse trails	kids	flora	bird-watching	fall foliage	historical sites	geographical features
URBAN-SUBURBAN MINNEAPOLIS *(continued)*								
15 Hyland Lake Park Reserve, Richardson Interpretive Trail	70				✓			
16 Lake Nokomis	74		✓					
17 Minnehaha Falls and Creek	78					✓	✓	✓
18 Mississippi Gorge Trail	82	✓					✓	✓
19 Rice Creek North Regional Trail	87	✓		✓				
20 Wood Lake Nature Center	91		✓		✓			
SOUTHWEST								
21 Cleary Lake Regional Park	98	✓	✓					
22 Douglas State Trail	102					✓		
23 Lake Byllesby Regional Park	105							
24 Louisville Swamp, Mazomani Trail	108		✓					
25 Minnesota Valley State Recreation Area, Lawrence Trail	113					✓	✓	✓
26 Murphy-Hanrehan Park Reserve	117						✓	✓
27 Sakatah Lake State Park	120							
SOUTHEAST								
28 Afton State Park	126		✓	✓	✓			✓
29 Barn Bluff	130				✓	✓	✓	✓
30 Cannon Valley Trail	134			✓	✓		✓	
31 Cottage Grove Ravine Regional Park	139				✓			✓
32 Frontenac State Park, Bluffside Trail	142		✓		✓	✓	✓	✓
33 Lebanon Hills Regional Park, Holland/Jensen Lakes Loop	146			✓	✓			✓
34 Miesville Ravine Park Reserve	151				✓			
35 Nerstrand–Big Woods State Park, Big Woods Trail	154	✓	✓		✓	✓	✓	✓
36 Spring Lake Park Reserve, Schaar's Bluff Trail	158				✓			

REGION Hike #/Hike name	page	multiuse trails	kids	flora	bird-watching	fall foliage	historical sites	geographical features
NORTHWEST								
37 Baker Park Reserve	164			✓	✓			
38 Baylor Regional Park	168	✓						
39 Carver Park Reserve/ Lowry Nature Center, Tamarack Trail	171							
40 Crow-Hassan Park Reserve	175		✓					
41 Elm Creek Park Reserve	179			✓				
42 Elm Creek Park Reserve, Eastman Nature Trail	183	✓	✓					
43 Lake Maria State Park	188				✓			✓
44 Lake Minnewashta Regional Park, Marsh Trail Loop	192							✓
45 Lake Rebecca Park Reserve	195							
46 Rum River Central Regional Park	199							
47 Rum River North County Park	203							
48 Sand Dunes State Forest, Ann Lake	206		✓			✓		✓
49 Sherburne National Wildlife Refuge, Prairie's Edge Trail	209			✓				
50 Snail Lake	213							
NORTHEAST								
51 Gateway State Trail	218							
52 Interstate State Park, Minnesota	222				✓		✓	
53 Interstate State Park, Wisconsin	226						✓	
54 Kinnickinnic State Park, Wisconsin	231							
55 Pine Point Regional Park Trail	234				✓			
56 Red Cedar State Trail, Wisconsin	238						✓	
57 Tamarack Nature Center	242							
58 Wild River State Park	245			✓				
59 William O'Brien State Park, Upper Park Trail	249			✓			✓	
60 Willow River State Park	253							

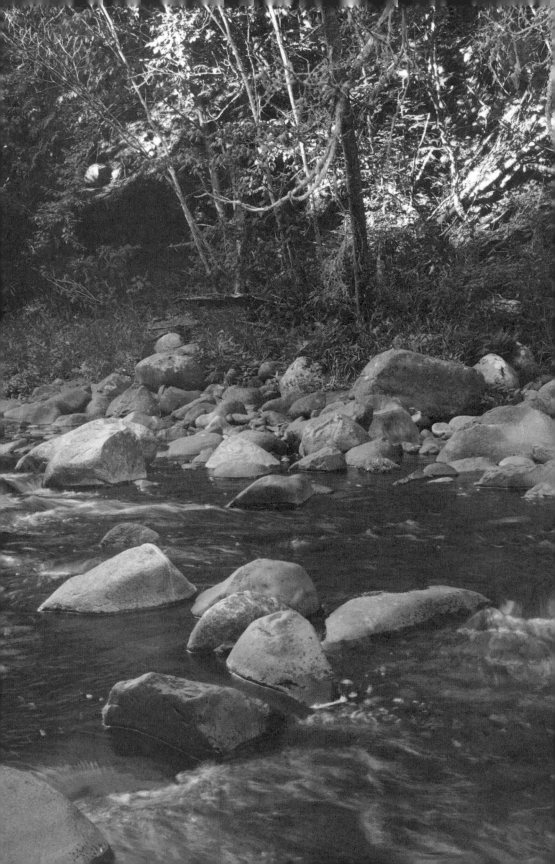

INTRODUCTION

60 Hikes within 60 Miles: Minneapolis and St. Paul, as the title suggests, offers hikers a descriptive glimpse of some of the best day-hiking trails within an hour's drive of downtown Minneapolis and St. Paul, Minnesota's Twin Cities. Interconnecting trail networks enable hikers to literally walk from one end of the metropolitan area to the other, all the while enjoying pockets of flora and fauna, including preserved or restored presettlement prairies and northern forests, that might otherwise go unnoticed.

If you're new to hiking or even if you're a seasoned trail-smith, take a few minutes to read the following introduction. It explains how this book is organized and how to use it, better enabling you to access the many splendid trail miles that await.

HOW TO USE THIS GUIDEBOOK

THE OVERVIEW MAP AND OVERVIEW-MAP KEY

Use the overview map on the inside front cover to assess the exact location of each hike's primary trailhead. Each hike's number appears on the overview map, on the map key facing the overview map, and in the table of contents. As you flip through the book, a hike's full profile is easy to locate by watching for the hike number at the top of each right-hand page.

REGIONAL MAPS

The book is divided into regions, and prefacing each regional section is an overview map. The regional maps provide more detail than the overview map, bringing you closer to the hike.

TRAIL MAPS

Each hike contains a detailed map that shows the trailhead, the route, significant features, facilities, and topographic

1

landmarks such as creeks, overlooks, and peaks. Each trailhead's GPS coordinates are included with each profile (see discussion below).

LEGEND

A legend that details the symbols found on trail maps appears on the inside back cover.

GPS TRAILHEAD COORDINATES

Readers can easily access all trailheads in this book by using the directions given, the overview map, and the trail map, which shows at least one major road leading into the area. But for those who enjoy using the latest GPS technology to navigate, the necessary data has been provided.

This book includes the GPS coordinates for each trailhead in latitude–longitude format. These numbers tell you where you are by locating a point east or west of the prime meridian that passes through Greenwich, England (longitude), and north or south of the equator (latitude).

For readers who own a GPS unit, whether handheld or in a vehicle, the latitude–longitude coordinates provided on the first page of each hike may be entered into the unit. Just make sure yours is set to navigate using the WGS84 datum. Now you can navigate directly to the trailhead.

Trailheads that begin at parking areas can be reached by car, but other hikes still require a short walk to reach the trailhead from a parking area. In those cases, a handheld GPS unit is necessary to continue the navigation process.

In this book, latitude–longitude coordinates are expressed in degrees and decimal minutes. For example, the coordinates for Hike 1, Battle Creek (page 18), are as follows: N92° 59.989'; W44° 56.032'. To convert GPS coordinates given in degrees, minutes, and seconds to the format shown above, divide the seconds by 60. For more on GPS technology, visit **usgs.gov.**

HIKE PROFILES

Each hike contains six key items: an In Brief description of the trail, a Key At-a-Glance Information box, directions to the trail, trailhead coordinates, a trail map, and a trail description. Combined, the maps and information provide a clear method to assess each trail from the comfort of your favorite chair.

IN BRIEF

A "taste of the trail." Think of this section as a snapshot focused on the historical landmarks, beautiful vistas, and other sights you might encounter on the hike.

KEY AT-A-GLANCE INFORMATION

The following information gives you a quick idea of the statistics and specifics of each hike:

LENGTH How long the trail is from start to finish. There may be options to shorten or extend the hikes, but the mileage corresponds to the described hike. Use the Description as a guide to customizing the hike for your ability or time constraints.

CONFIGURATION A description of what the trail might look like from overhead. Trails can be loops, out-and-backs (trails on which one enters and leaves along the same path), point to points, figure eights, or a combination of shapes.

DIFFICULTY Estimates the degree of effort an average hiker should expect on a given hike. I have used familiar terms and explained in the Preface my personal preference for leisurely hiking.

SCENERY A short summary of the hike's attractions and what to expect in terms of plant life, wildlife, natural wonders, and historical features.

EXPOSURE A quick check of how much sun you can expect on your shoulders during the hike. Descriptions are self-explanatory and include terms such as "shady," "exposed," and "sunny."

TRAFFIC Indicates how busy the trail might be on an average day. Trail traffic, of course, varies from day to day and season to season. Weekend days typically see the most visitors.

TRAIL SURFACE Indicates whether the trail is paved, rocky, gravel, dirt, boardwalk, or a mixture of surfaces.

HIKING TIME Tells how long it took me to hike the trail. A slow but steady hiker will average 2–3 miles an hour, depending on the terrain.

SEASON Time(s) of year when the hike is accessible.

ACCESS A notation of any necessary fees or permits required to access the trail or park at the trailhead.

MAPS Lists which maps are useful, in my opinion, for this hike and where to find them.

FACILITIES What you can expect in terms of restrooms and water at the trailhead or nearby.

SPECIAL COMMENTS Provides you with those little extra details that don't fit into any of the above categories. Here you'll find reminders about such matters as park or road gate closings that could trap you or your car, trails that are susceptible to flooding, and hunting seasons that could affect your hiking.

CONTACT Gives you contact information, including phone number and website, in case you want to do additional research.

DIRECTIONS

Used with the overview map, the driving directions will help you locate each trailhead. Once you've reached the trailhead, park only in designated areas.

GPS TRAILHEAD COORDINATES

The trailhead coordinates can be used in addition to the driving directions if you enter the coordinates into your GPS unit before you set out. See page 2 for more information.

DESCRIPTION

This is the heart of each hike. Here, I summarize the trail's essence and highlight any special traits the hike has to offer. The route is clearly outlined, including any landmarks, side trips, and possible alternate routes along the way. Ultimately, the Description will help you choose which hikes are best for you.

NEARBY ACTIVITIES

Look here for information on nearby dining, recreational opportunities, or other activities to fill out your day.

WEATHER

Minnesota's weather makes no exceptions for the Twin Cities. It can make you both unsuspectingly confident about sunshine and warmth and a worried second-guesser, all within a matter of hours. Dressing in layers is always a good plan. Even during spectacularly sunny weather, bringing a waterproof windbreaker is good comfort insurance against a cool lake breeze or persistent drizzle from a renegade rain cloud.

Four distinct seasons, each with attitude, present almost every form of weather imaginable through the course of a year.

Hiking in the Twin Cities can be done year-round on many of the trails, most of the time. Exceptions are during unseasonably cold or excessively snowy weather. Some summer hiking trails become cross-country skiing routes when winter sets in. Other trails can be used for winter hiking and snowshoeing.

While most trails mentioned in this book offer their amenities and attractions throughout the year, those that are particularly enjoyable during a certain season are noted in their profiles.

Early spring and late fall are especially nice times to hike in areas with dense understory, because less foliage means you can see deeper into the woods. Of course, hiking under a thick summer canopy of lush leaves or strolling through flaming fall colors is cause enough to try these trails several times a year.

AVERAGE DAILY TEMPERATURE BY MONTH: MINNEAPOLIS AND ST. PAUL, MN						
	JAN	FEB	MAR	APR	MAY	JUN
HIGH	20°F	26°F	39°F	56°F	69°F	78°F
LOW	2°F	9°F	22°F	36°F	47°F	57°F

AVERAGE DAILY TEMPERATURE BY MONTH: MINNEAPOLIS AND ST. PAUL, MN						
	JUL	AUG	SEP	OCT	NOV	DEC
HIGH	84°F	80°F	70°F	58°F	41°F	25°F
LOW	63°F	60°F	50°F	38°F	25°F	10°F

Average lows and highs range from 2°F to 20°F in January to 63°F to 84°F in July. The heaviest monthly rainfall occurs between May (above 2 inches) and September (above 2.5 inches), peaking at about 4 inches in July. The average humidity for this region between May and September is about 53%.

ECOLOGICAL REGIONS

There are three main ecological regions in Minnesota: northern conifers (also called Pinelands), hardwood forests, and prairies. Two of these regions, the Pinelands and hardwoods, converge very close to the Twin Cities. Many of the Twin Cities and surrounding suburban area parks feature the aspen, birch, spruce, pine, and fir forests that make up the majority of the Pinelands region. Coupled with the lakes, bogs, and wildlife associated with such environments, these parks offer hikers an opportunity to experience the type of ecological flora and fauna common to the state's northern regions.

The prairies of Minnesota, which once covered vast portions of Minnesota and millions of acres of the Great Plains, are now preserved in small sections and plots through this region. Many of the hikes in this book include routes through or around reestablished prairie systems within a park or preserve.

AREA GEOLOGY

There are four main geological areas that converge at the Twin Cities: The Big Woods—made up of mixed hardwoods that virtually covered the eastern half of Minnesota before settlements encroached from the east—dominate the western portions of the Twin Cities as well as a few major remnants to the south. The St. Croix moraines are glacial deposits left over from the most recent ice age. Much of the landscape east of St. Paul has been sculpted into reminders of the great sheet of ice that once covered the area. To the north of the Twin Cities lie the great sand plains of Anoka. Jack pine forests dominate this area. The oak savannas of the southern portion of the Twin Cities region are reminders of the vastness of the prairies and plains that once covered the entire Midwest. The savannas, with their rolling hills, island of oaks and other hardwoods, and pockets of open prairielike cover, are slowly being brought back in many of the parks through prairie-restoration projects, some of which are mentioned in association with particular hikes in this book.

WATER

How much is enough? Well, one simple physiological fact should persuade you to err on the side of excess when deciding how much water to pack: a hiker working hard in 90°F heat needs about 10 quarts of fluid per day. That's 2.5 gallons—12 large water bottles or 16 small ones. In other words, pack one or two bottles even for short hikes.

While it's no problem to carry adequate supplies of water on these day hikes, some hikers and backpackers hit the trail prepared to purify water found along the route. This method, while less dangerous than drinking untreated water, comes with risks if not properly performed. Purifiers with ceramic filters are the safest. Many hikers pack the slightly distasteful tetraglycine–hydroperiodide tablets to debug water (sold under the names Potable Aqua, Coughlan's, and others). Aquamira chlorine dioxide tablets are nearly tasteless and almost weightless; gravity filters and hydration systems with inline filters are convenient and effective as well. SteriPEN is an ultraviolet-light treatment device that weighs about 10 ounces. If none of these methods is available, bringing the water to a boil is enough to kill the pathogens.

Probably the most common waterborne bug that hikers face is giardia, which may not hit until one to four weeks after ingestion. It will have you living in the bathroom, passing noxious rotten-egg gas, vomiting, and shivering with chills. Other parasites to worry about include *E. coli* and *cryptosporidium,* both of which are harder to kill than giardia.

For most people, the pleasures of hiking make carrying water a relatively minor price to pay to remain healthy. If you're tempted to drink "found water," do so only if you understand the risks involved. Better yet, hydrate before your hike, carry (and drink) 6 ounces of water for every mile you plan to hike, and hydrate after the hike. If in an emergency situation you find yourself having to choose between drinking untreated water and getting dehydrated, by all means drink it—if you get sick, see a doctor after your rescue.

CLOTHING

For most hikes in the summer season, your choice of trail clothing can vary widely and is really more a matter of personal preference. Shorts or long pants? Long-sleeve or short-sleeve shirt? Those are probably decisions you'll make the morning of the hike without much thought. For longer, more strenuous hikes, you may want to consider synthetic moisture-wicking fabric instead of the trusty cotton T-shirt that retains moisture and can even lead to hypothermia if the temperature drops quickly. It's a good idea to pack a lightweight fleece or an extra outer layer for higher elevations or in case there is a surprise drop in temperature.

When it comes to footwear, comfort and personal preference should be your guide. Since these are all day hikes and don't require a heavy pack, you may find that a lightweight trail shoe is your best bet. Tennis shoes may be sufficient for paved trails and short hikes of less than 3 miles. For longer hikes and those involving steep, rocky terrain, you'll want to consider a hiking shoe that has a thicker, firmer sole that offers more support.

Proper footwear is absolutely essential. Gripping soles and solid ankle support are mandatory—even on groomed or paved pathways. A properly worn-in boot or hiking shoe should be used, especially on longer hikes. Breaking in a stiff pair of trekking shoes on even a short hike can breed a crop of blisters.

A wide-brimmed hat to protect against the sun or rain and a lightweight rain jacket or windbreaker may be handy, too.

ESSENTIAL EQUIPMENT

One of the first rules of hiking is to be prepared for anything. The simplest way to be prepared is to carry the essentials. In addition to carrying the following items, you need to know how to use them, especially navigation items. Always consider worst-case scenarios such as getting lost, hiking back in the dark, broken gear (for example, a broken hip strap on your pack or a water filter getting plugged), twisting an ankle, or a brutal thunderstorm. The items listed here don't cost a lot of money, don't take up much room in a pack, and don't weigh much, but they might just save your life.

EMERGENCY TOOLS: Signal whistle, signal mirror, knife, multitool, cord

EXTRA CLOTHING: Insulation layer, gloves, rain gear, socks, soft-shell jacket

FOOD: Nutrition bars, snacks, or meals for the day, plus extra; always try to return with some food.

FIRE: Matches, lighter, fire starter, or stove with full fuel bottle/canister

FIRST-AID KIT: With fresh supplies, instructions, and the knowledge to use them

LIGHT: Headlamp with fresh batteries

MAP AND COMPASS: Trail or topographic map, simple compass, route description, and the knowledge to use them

SUN PROTECTION: Hat, sunglasses, sunscreen, lip balm

SHELTER: A space blanket or Siltarp can provide immediate sun or rain protection for accident victims.

TREKKING POLES: In addition to keeping your footing steady, they can act as a third leg, monopod, shelter pole, cougar and bear defense, poison-oak deflector, or handy implement for poking and irritating creatures while dawdling.

WATER: Full bottles, plus extra, or water-treatment tablets/purifying filter

This list is fully weather- and trip-dependent. The list will help you structure and plan for the requirements of each trip.

No matter where you go, though, it's a good idea to consider other, non-essential gear that could add to your experience, comfort, or general pleasure on the trail.

FIRST-AID KIT

A typical kit may contain more items than you think necessary. The following are just the basics. Prepackaged kits in waterproof bags are available (Atwater Carey and Adventure Medical make a variety of kits). Even though there are quite a few items listed here, they pack down into a small space.

Ace bandages or Spenco joint wraps

Adhesive bandages

Antibiotic ointment (Neosporin or the generic equivalent)

Aspirin or acetaminophen

Benadryl or the generic equivalent, diphenhydramine (in case of allergic reactions)

Butterfly-closure bandages

Epinephrine in a prefilled syringe (for people known to have severe allergic reactions to such things as bee stings)

Gauze (one roll and a half dozen 4-by-4-inch compress pads)

Hydrogen peroxide or iodine

Insect repellent

Moleskin/Spenco Second Skin

WHAT TO BRING

Besides a camera bag, none of these trails should necessitate carrying anything more than a fanny pack or day pack. Adequate water for your metabolism and thirst-quenching needs should be carried at all times. Most of the areas provide water, either at the trailhead, along some trails, or at the visitor center/park headquarters.

Fuel in the form of snacks—such as energy bars or trail mix—is a personal preference. Personally, I like the idea of stopping at a particularly scenic overlook along a trail and having a snack while my other senses feast on all the stimuli surrounding me.

Equally important, from my perspective, is to bring along a notebook or journal to record what you see, sketch what you observe, and describe what you think or feel along the trail. This and a good guidebook can expand your level of appreciation for all that surrounds you during each hike.

HIKING WITH CHILDREN

No one is too young for a nice hike in the woods or through a city park. Flat, short, and shaded trails are best with an infant. Toddlers who have not quite mastered walking can still tag along, riding on an adult's back in a child carrier.

Children who are walking can, of course, follow along with an adult. Use common sense to judge a child's capacity to hike a particular trail. Always plan for the possibility that the child will tire quickly and have to be carried. When packing for the hike, remember the child's needs as well as your own. Make sure children are adequately clothed for the weather, have proper shoes, and are properly protected from the sun with sunscreen and clothing. Kids dehydrate quickly, so make sure you have plenty of clean water or other drinks for everyone.

Depending on age, ability, and hike difficulty, most children should enjoy some of the short hikes described in this book. Hikes suitable for children are noted in the chart on pages xvii–xix.

THE BUSINESS HIKER

Whether you live in or near the Twin Cities area, are here on business, or are just traveling through as a casual visitor, these hikes are the perfect opportunity to make a quick getaway from the demands of commerce. Some of the hikes are located close to government buildings and other office areas classified as urban and are easily accessed from downtown areas.

Instead of grabbing a burger down the street, pack a lunch and head for a nearby trail—the local and state parklands are a good bet—to take a relaxing break from the office or that tiresome convention. Or plan ahead and take along a small group of your business comrades. A well-planned half-day getaway is the perfect complement to a business stay in the Twin Cities metropolitan area.

GENERAL SAFETY

Dangerous situations can occur outdoors, but as long as you use sound judgment and prepare yourself before hitting the trail, you'll be much safer in the woods than in most urban areas of the country. It's better to look at a backcountry hike as a fascinating chance to discover the unknown rather than a setting for potential disaster. These tips will help make your trip safer and easier.

- **Always carry food and water, whether you're planning to go overnight or not. Food will give you energy, help keep you warm, and sustain you in an emergency until help arrives. You never know if you'll have a stream nearby when you become thirsty. Bring potable water, or treat water before drinking it from a stream or other source.**

- **Stay on designated trails. Most hikers get lost when they leave the path. Even on the most clearly marked trails, you usually reach a point where you have to stop and consider which way to go. If you become disoriented, don't panic. As soon as you think you may be off-track, stop, assess your current direction, and then retrace your steps back to the point where you went awry. Using a map, a compass, and this book—and keeping in mind what you've passed thus far—reorient yourself and trust your judgment about which way to go. If you become absolutely unsure of that, return to your vehicle the way you came in. Should you become completely lost and have no idea how to return to the trailhead, remaining in place along the trail and waiting for help is most often the best option for adults and always the best option for children.**

- **Be especially careful when crossing streams. Whether you're fording the stream or crossing on a log, make every step count. If you're not sure you can maintain your balance on a foot log, go ahead and ford the stream instead.**

When fording a stream, use a trekking pole or stout stick for balance, and face upstream as you cross. If a stream seems too deep to ford, turn back. Whatever is on the other side isn't worth risking your life for.

- Be careful at overlooks. While these areas may provide spectacular views, they are potentially hazardous. Stay back from the edge of outcrops, and be absolutely sure of your footing.

- Standing dead trees and storm-damaged living trees pose a real hazard to hikers and tent campers. These trees may have loose or broken limbs that could fall at any time. When choosing a resting spot or a backcountry campsite, look up.

- Know the symptoms of heat exhaustion. Excessive sweating, faintness, dizziness, clammy skin, vomiting, and paleness are all common symptoms. If symptoms arise, remove extra clothing, move to the shade, and drink plenty of water.

- Likewise, know the symptoms of hypothermia. Shivering and forgetfulness are the two most common indicators of this insidious killer. Hypothermia can occur at any elevation, even in the summer, especially when the hiker is wearing lightweight cotton clothing. Get the victim shelter, warm liquids if conscious, and dry clothes or a dry sleeping bag.

- Bring your brain. A cool, calculating mind is the single most important piece of equipment you'll need on the trail. Think before you act. Watch your step. Plan ahead. Avoiding accidents before they happen is the best recipe for a rewarding and relaxing hike.

- Ask questions. Forest and park employees are there to help. It's a lot easier to gain advice beforehand and avoid a mishap away from civilization when it's too late to amend an error. Use your head out there.

ANIMAL AND PLANT HAZARDS

SNAKES

Most of the snakes found in the Twin Cities area are nonvenomous. However, two species, the timber rattlesnake and the massasauga, have been spotted here—specifically in the southeasternmost section of the state.

Always give rattlesnakes plenty of space and never approach one on purpose. Rattlesnakes prefer warmth but not searing heat. They are most active during spring and around dusk. Their favorite hangouts are rock crevices, tall brush, and under shady branches. Vigilantly watch your step while hiking, and peer over any rock outcrops first before touching them.

TICKS

You can use several strategies to reduce your chances of getting ticks embedded in your skin. Some people choose to wear light-colored clothing, so ticks can be spotted before they make it to the skin. Insect repellent containing DEET is known as an effective deterrent. Most important, though, be sure to inspect your-self visually at the end of a hike. During your post-hike shower, take a moment to do a more complete body check. For ticks that are already embedded, removal with tweezers is best.

MOSQUITOES

While not a common occurrence, individuals can become infected with the West Nile virus from the bite of an infected mosquito. Culex mosquitoes, the primary varieties that can transmit West Nile virus to humans, thrive in urban rather than wilderness areas. They lay their eggs in stagnant water and can breed in any stand-ing water that remains for more than five days. Most people infected with West Nile virus have no symptoms of illness, but some may become ill, usually 3–15 days after being bitten.

Most at risk are the elderly and those with weakened immune systems. Though the risk of infection is relatively low, hikers should consider taking mea-sures to prevent mosquito bites. Remedies include using insect repellent and wear-ing clothes that completely cover the arms and legs.

POISON IVY

Poison ivy is ever present in the region's forested parks as well as alongside trails in both country and urban settings. It can be a small, unimposing plant or a taller shrublike bush. Learning to recognize it by its distinct three-lobed compound leaf will reward you many times over during the summer and fall.

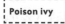
Poison ivy

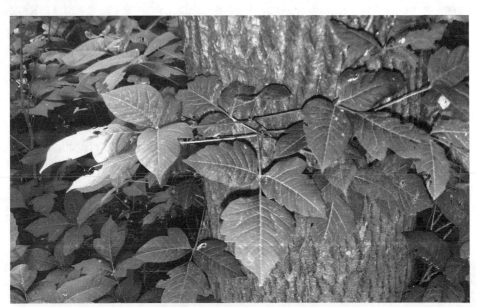

Usually within 12–14 hours of exposure (but sometimes much later), raised lines and/or blisters will appear, accompanied by a terrible itch. Refrain from scratching because bacteria under your fingernails can cause infection and spread the rash to other parts of your body. Wash and dry the rash thoroughly, applying calamine lotion or another product to help dry the rash. If itching or blistering is severe, seek medical attention. Remember that oil-contaminated clothes, pets, or hiking gear can easily spread the rash to you or someone else, so wash not only any exposed parts of your body but also clothes, gear, and pets.

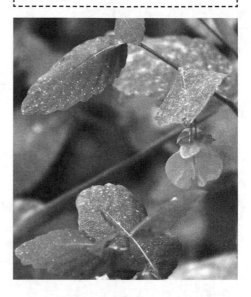

Jewelweed, a plant that counters the effects of poison ivy

STINGING NETTLE

Another nasty plant, stinging nettle, can produce a burn similar to that of a jellyfish or other skin-irritating plants and animals. Learn to identify this tall, tooth-edged leafy plant as well.

PRICKLY MOUNTAIN ASH

While several species of shrubs, such as the woody hawthorn and the more vine-like raspberry, have thorns, none compare to the prickly mountain ash. Growing unassumingly along the trail, looking innocently like a small green ash, the prickly ash has needle-sharp thorns ready to bite the hand that grabs it or lash out at an arm or leg that passes too closely.

ENJOY THE EXPERIENCE

What all these trails have in common is an opportunity to turn a part of your day into a stroll in the park smack-dab in the middle of the city. For some of us, a hike is a brisk walk for exercise; for others it's a leisurely paced traipse through unexplored woods. Sometimes it's a planned trek of discovery with the goal perhaps to add a new bird to your life list or catch your favorite wildflower at peak bloom. Whatever the inspiration, the trails in this book are pathways to other activities, observations, and pleasures.

Of course, don't litter and don't remove things that others might enjoy. Collect images mentally or with a camera or sketch pad. Whether yours is the path less taken or the one deeply worn, enjoy each as though you were the first to lay foot upon it. Treat the place with care, as if it were your own backyard.

TOPO MAPS

The maps in this book have been produced with great care and, used with the hiking directions, will direct you to the trails and help you stay on course. However, you will find superior detail and valuable information in the USGS's 7.5-minute-series topographic maps. One well-known free topo service on the Web is **Microsoft Research Maps (msrmaps.com)**. Online services such as **Trails.com** charge annual fees for additional features such as shaded relief, which makes the topography stand out more. If you expect to print out many topo maps each year, it might be worth paying for such extras. The downside to USGS topos is that most are outdated, having been created 20–30 years ago. But they still provide excellent topographic detail.

Digital topographic-map programs, such as DeLorme's Topo USA, enable you to review topo maps of the entire United States on your computer. Data gathered while hiking with a GPS unit can be downloaded into the software, letting you plot your own hikes. Of course, Google Earth (**earth.google.com**) does away with topo maps and their inaccuracies, replacing them with satellite imagery and its inaccuracies. Regardless, what one lacks, the other augments. Google Earth is an excellent tool whether or not you have difficulty with topos. Getting a quick set of eyes on the ground can be invaluable when you're planning your hike.

If you're new to hiking, you might be wondering, "What's a topographic map?" In short, a topo indicates not only linear distance but elevation as well, using contour lines. These lines spread across the map like dozens of intricate spiderwebs. Each line represents a particular elevation, and at the base of each topo, a contour's interval designation is given. If the contour interval is 20 feet, then the distance between each contour line is 20 feet. Follow five contour lines up on the same map, and the elevation has increased by 100 feet.

Let's assume that the 7.5-minute-series topo reads "contour interval 40 feet," that the short trail we'll be hiking is 2 inches in length on the map, and that it crosses five contour lines from beginning to end. What do we know? Well, because the linear scale of this series is 2,000 feet to the inch (roughly 2.75 inches representing 1 mile), we know that our trail is about three-fourths of a mile long (2 inches equals 4,000 feet). But we also know we'll be climbing or descending 200 vertical feet (five contour lines are 40 feet each) over that distance. And the elevation designations written on occasional contour lines will tell us if we're heading up or down.

In addition to outdoors shops and bike shops, other places in the Twin Cities metro area likely to carry topos are major universities and some public libraries, where you may be able to photocopy the ones you need and avoid the cost of buying them. If you want your own and can't find them locally, visit The USGS Store (**store.usgs.gov**).

TRAIL ETIQUETTE

Whether you're on a city walk or on a long hike, remember that great care and resources (from nature as well as from tax dollars) have gone into creating the trails and paths you're enjoying. Taking care of them begins with you, the hiker. Treat the trail, wildlife, flora, and your fellow hikers with respect. Here are a few general ideas to keep in mind while hiking:

1. **HIKE ON OPEN TRAILS ONLY.** Respect trail and road closures (ask if you're not sure), avoid trespassing on private land, and obtain any required permits or authorization. Leave gates as you found them or as marked.

2. **LEAVE NO TRACE** of your visit other than footprints. Be sensitive to the land beneath your feet. This also means staying on the trail and not creating any new trails. Be sure to pack out what you pack in. No one likes to see trash someone else has left behind.

3. **NEVER SPOOK ANIMALS.** An unannounced approach, a sudden movement, or a loud noise can startle them. A surprised animal can be dangerous to you, others, and itself. Give animals plenty of space.

4. **PLAN AHEAD.** Know your equipment, your ability, and the area where you are hiking—and prepare accordingly. Be self-sufficient at all times; carry necessary supplies (such as ample water, sunscreen, and insect repellent) for changes in weather or other conditions. A well-executed trip is a satisfaction to you and not a burden or offense to others.

5. **BE COURTEOUS** to other hikers, bikers, and all people you meet while hiking.

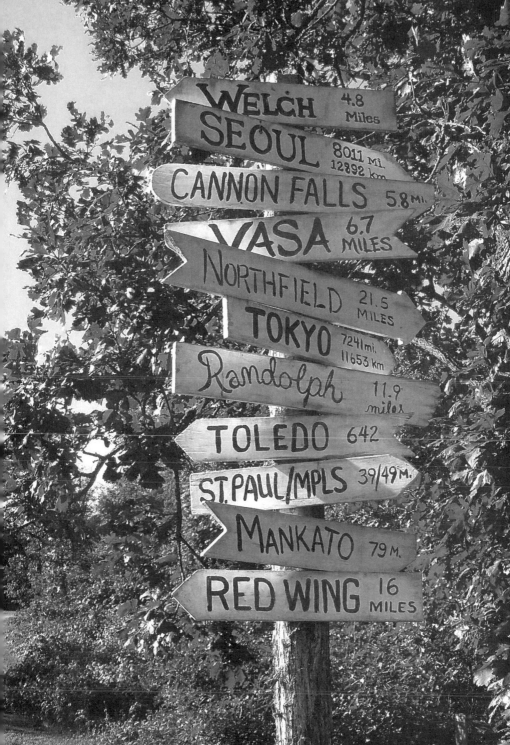

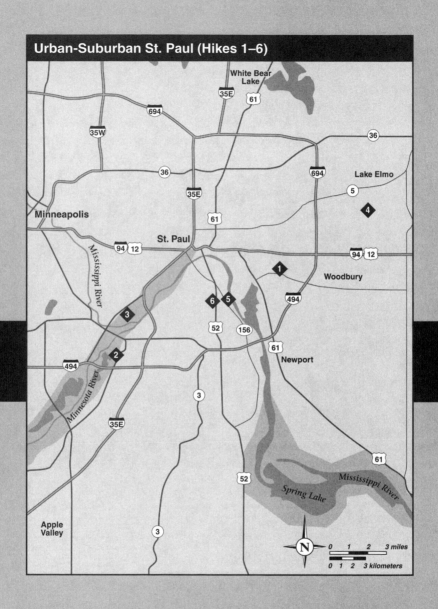

Urban-Suburban St. Paul (Hikes 1–6)

White Bear Lake

35E · 61

694

35W

35E

36

694 · Lake Elmo

5

4

36

35E

61

Minneapolis

Mississippi River

94 · 12

St. Paul

94 · 12

1

Woodbury

6 · 5

494

52

156

3

61

Newport

2

494

Minnesota River

3

35E

61

52

Spring Lake

Mississippi River

Apple Valley

3

N

0   1   2   3 miles

0 1 2 3 kilometers

URBAN–SUBURBAN ST. PAUL

1 BATTLE CREEK

KEY AT-A-GLANCE INFORMATION

LENGTH: 4.4 miles

CONFIGURATION: Irregular circle

DIFFICULTY: Mostly easy walking with some gradual slopes

SCENERY: Impressive considering its city location; broad meadows and mature forests

EXPOSURE: Mixture of sun and shade

TRAFFIC: Lots of bike riders and hikers on evenings and weekends

TRAIL SURFACE: Paved throughout

HIKING TIME: 1.5–2 hours

SEASON: Year-round; some segments are designated ski trails in winter or serve as corridors to many spurs off main route.

ACCESS: No fees

MAPS: None; trailside map is slightly confusing; stay on paved bike/hike path

FACILITIES: None

SPECIAL COMMENTS: This trail has lots of birds and a large variety of trees for a city park.

CONTACT: Ramsey County Parks, (651) 748-2500

GPS TRAILHEAD COORDINATES

Latitude   N92° 59.989'

Longitude   W44° 56.032'

IN BRIEF

The southern unit has the best hiking within this multiunit park. Mature stands of hardwoods, small ponds nestled in among the trees, and winding paved paths that dip and climb gently through woods and meadows offer hikers a pleasant, woodsy setting right in the heart of southwest St. Paul.

DESCRIPTION

There are three distinct units to Battle Creek Park. The northern unit is made up of a picnic area, playgrounds, and other amenities centered on a small lake; the western unit is a trailhead at the end of the ravine through which Battle Creek flows; and the southern unit is a spaghetti network of trails through mature oaks and around the marsh—and the source of our hike of choice.

Begin at the parking lot off Lower Afton Road. At the far end of the lot are a trailhead for the Pet Trail on the left and a trailhead sign for the bike/hike trail that parallels the parking lot. The sign shows the trails, but the information is more confusing than helpful. There are no maps for Battle Creek of a scale or in sufficient detail to do any good, so the simple rule for this hike is to stay on the paved trail. There is only one intersection where this rule is challenged. Therefore, note a second rule: always take the paved trail to the left.

Directions

Head east on I-94, through St. Paul, to McKnight Road, and turn right (south) toward Lower Afton Road. Turn left (east) on Lower Afton Road; at 200 yards you'll come to the entrance to parking lot on the left.

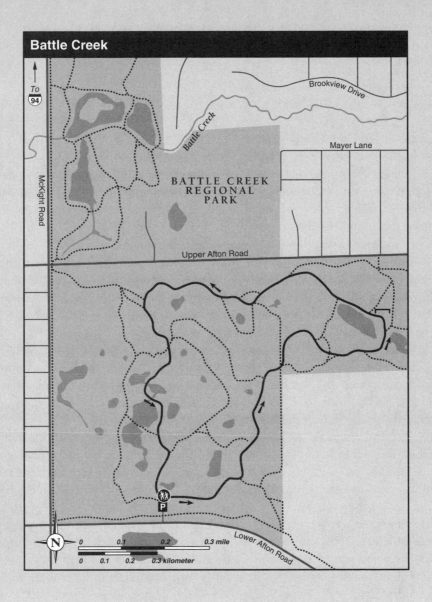

Battle Creek

BATTLE CREEK
REGIONAL
PARK

Brookview Drive

Mayer Lane

McKight Road

Battle Creek

To 94

Upper Afton Road

Lower Afton Road

N

0   0.1   0.2   0.3 mile

0   0.1   0.2   0.3 kilometer

Head uphill on the paved trail to the right of the bike/hike sign to begin the hike. As you start up the hill, you pass through typical upland forest species: oaks and ashes, a few scattered pine trees, and a modest understory of saplings and ground vegetation. These trails constantly meander around and through the woods, rising and dipping on a route that follows the rolling contours of the park.

The trail turns to the left into a denser stand of trees. A grass trail to the right is one of many you will encounter along this route—if you do happen upon a map, many of these trails are not marked, or are marked incorrectly. However, these are all ski trails and, as such, are not paved. An adventurous hiker can choose to add these trails and create additional loops to expand the hike. All eventually lead back to the main paved trail loop.

Continue on the paved section, past another grassy trail on the left, and through a mature stand of stately oaks. The trail will continue to meander and rise to an intersection of several trails. One is a utility corridor along a row of pine trees. No matter; stay on the paved trail past this intersection and follow the main trail to the left. Immediately past the intersection, circle around the bottom edge of a huge meadow covered in tall grass and wildflowers.

The trail skirts the southern edge of the meadow and then cuts to the right, through the middle of the expansive rolling meadow and down into a small stand of trees, mostly box elders. Trails will approach from both the right and the left, but keep in mind the rule to stay on the paved path, and it will lead you right down through the islands of trees and along a marshy area on the left.

You are now at the eastern end of the meadow, and the woods rise to your right as the path swings back to the left (north) and around the marshy area. Just before you come to another paved pathway on your right, you'll pass a small pond on the right. This is a good bird-viewing area where you can spot ducks, egrets, and possibly a great blue heron.

The intersection offers a paved path to the right heading over the crest of the meadow's edge. Stick to the path straight ahead (the left fork), and continue around the marsh rushes and grasses. About 100 yards along this open section of the trail you'll come to a bench flanked by two cottonwoods—giants by any standard—towering over the trail.

The trail enters the woods again as it ascends and descends with the rolling terrain. You will wind through a stand of hardwoods before coming out at another main intersection. This is actually a northern trailhead for this section of the park and is adjacent to the tennis courts. A couple of paved paths lead off to the right at this point, but you want to stay on the leftmost trail to head back into the wooded area. There is a trailhead sign with trails designated, but, like the sign at the southern end, its information is not very clear. From here to the end of the trail, the paved section is the main route and remains easy to follow.

For the next mile the trail dips and winds in a series of S turns through a lowland section of the park. You will cross two major intersections, both grass, before winding through a bog area composed of a couple of small ponds, one on each side of the trail. The path cuts sharply to the left and then sharply to the right as it swings and dips past these two wet areas.

You emerge into an open understory beneath tall maples and box elders before the path rises again as it goes into the final upland wooded area. Another small pond on the left marks the end of the trail as the path opens onto the clearing at the start of the trailhead at the end of the parking lot.

NEARBY ACTIVITIES

Hike through the western section of Battle Creek up a rocky ravine and through the forested area on the bluffs. Park at the Point Douglas Street parking lot off US 61. Indian Mounds Park, 2 miles to the west, offers short trails and native history.

BIG RIVERS REGIONAL TRAIL 2

IN BRIEF

More than half the river distance of this trail is laid out atop an embankment that supports railroad tracks routed along the Minnesota and Mississippi rivers. Vistas of the river below are embellished by wildflowers along the trail and periodic glimpses of barges, motorboats, and even a paddle wheeler or two plying the waters.

DESCRIPTION

The official trailhead for this trail is actually at the northern terminus at Lilydale. However, because of very limited parking, a rather unsafe road crossing, and the fact that the southern end is better developed in all those regards, I describe the hike leaving from a major trail juncture at the southern end of this particular section.

The Big Rivers Regional Trail is part of the extensive Dakota County Parks system that offers St. Paulites and visitors many opportunities to enjoy the outdoor amenities available throughout much of the southern St. Paul metropolitan area. This trail is just a little bit south and east of downtown and gives

----

Directions ⟶

SOUTH TRAILHEAD: From south Minneapolis, take MN 55 south to Mendota Heights Road. Turn right and go about 0.5 mile to CR 31. Continue past CR 31 for 0.25 mile to the south trailhead parking lot.

NORTH TRAILHEAD/SHUTTLE POINT: From the parking lot at the south trailhead, go north on MN 13 about 3.75 miles to Lilydale Road. Turn left (west) and drive about 0.1 mile to parking area just before road goes under railroad overpass.

KEY AT-A-GLANCE INFORMATION

LENGTH: 3.9–7.9 miles

CONFIGURATION: Point to point or out-and-back

DIFFICULTY: Easy

SCENERY: Mostly vistas of the Minnesota and Mississippi rivers through openings in the trees along their banks

EXPOSURE: Sunny throughout, with little shade

TRAFFIC: Multiuse trail especially popular with bicyclists

TRAIL SURFACE: Paved throughout

HIKING TIME: 1.5–3 hours

SEASON: Year-round

ACCESS: No fees for trail use or parking

MAPS: At trailheads or at dakotacounty.net/parks

FACILITIES: Information kiosk and vault toilet at each end; no facilities along trail

SPECIAL COMMENTS: You'll get a bird's-eye view of the Minnesota and Mississippi rivers from the railroad track embankment above, all while staying close to downtown St. Paul.

CONTACT: (651) 437-3191

GPS TRAILHEAD COORDINATES

SOUTH TRAILHEAD:
Latitude   N93° 10.413'
Longitude   W44° 52.035'

NORTH TRAILHEAD:
Latitude   N93° 8.107'
Longitude   W44° 54.281'

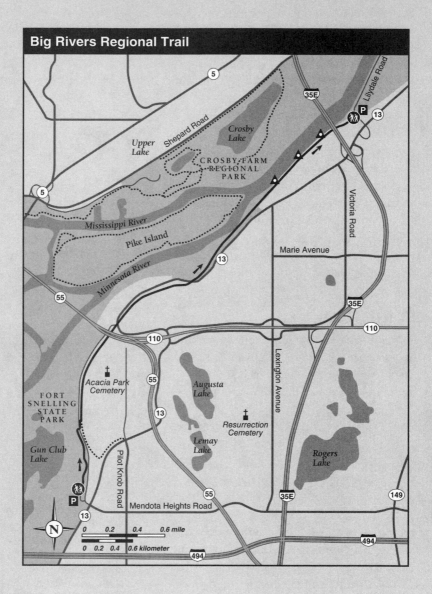

Big Rivers Regional Trail

hikers a chance to experience both the Minnesota and the Mississippi rivers from a unique perspective—a bird's-eye view from the train tracks!

Built on the bed of the Minnesota Central Railroad, the trail follows a fairly straight and level course between limestone bluff tops and the tree-lined banks of the rivers below. Historically speaking, this trail features a lofty view of Fort Snelling and the confluence of the Minnesota and Mississippi rivers—a strategic location both politically and commercially. Pike Island (see the profile for the Fort Snelling State Park hike on page 67, too) is the site of important negotiations between nonnative settlers and the original inhabitants of this area, the Sioux.

There are three key points to remember about this and other regional trails that are routed along a former railroad bed: First, they are designed to be multiuse, which means you'll share the trail with others, mostly bicyclists; second, no motorized vehicles are allowed; and third, since trails are old train routes, there are no loops or cutoffs to bring you back to the start along another route. These are straight-line trails that start in one location and end several miles down the trail. In the case of the Big Rivers Regional Trail, there are a few places along the way you can intercept the trail and take off either north or south along the route. To return to your starting point, you either have to reverse direction and rehike the same trail or arrange to be picked up or have a car shuttle worked out in advance.

Starting at the parking lot at the end of Mendota Heights Road, from the overlook you can get a sense of the breadth of the Minnesota River Valley just before the river joins up with the Mississippi about 1.5 miles north. There is also a small picnic area and a vault toilet. There are no facilities out on the trail.

Maps of the trail are available from a mailbox on a post next to the information bulletin board at the edge of the parking lot. From here this hike heads north along an 8-foot-wide paved trail, through a stand of majestic cottonwoods; it winds through this forest for about 0.5 mile. Once you come out of the wooded area, you'll cross MN 13 and will continue north on the other side of this highway for about 0.75 mile.

This section parallels the highway along a slight climb in elevation to the underpasses of MN 55 and MN 110 at about mile 1.2. This is the intersection with Victoria Curve and could be a shuttle point if you wanted to concentrate on only the northern two-thirds of this hike. Once the trail starts back down a gentle drop in elevation, you begin to hike past the backs of houses and businesses in the community of Mendota Heights.

As you approach the D Street intersection, the trail widens to a full city-street's width for about 100 yards while passing behind the commercial section of this community. This is your first opportunity to actually see the old railroad bed upon which this section of the trail is laid. Houses to your right are at the bottom of a steep 30-foot embankment, while the backs of stores on your left are only about 10 feet below the trail's surface.

Continuing north, the trail crosses the highway again at about mile 2. An unmarked gravel parking area just to the left of this crossing seems to be an unofficial parking lot for trail users—another shuttle drop-off to keep in mind. Once you cross the highway, the trail gets really exciting because you are approaching the river bluffs, where the trail above finally meets up with the train tracks below.

At first there is little to indicate that you are now above the river, because of the thick foliage lining both sides of the trail. This lush corridor is mostly under-story vegetation with some taller trees such as ironwood and box elder. When I hiked this trail in May, there were pleasing patches of wild roses in bloom right along the edge of the trail.

The trail is laid out about 30 feet below the top edge of the limestone bluffs that form the rim of the river valley in this area. Occasionally there is a break in the vegetation, and large knobs and walls of yellowish limestone are exposed overhead. There are ledges, deep cuts, and even narrow recesses that look like cave entrances appearing randomly along this trail.

The river comes into view below the trail as the pathway approaches the railroad tracks below. At first the tracks are at least 20 to 30 feet below the trail. Eventually they are within about 10 feet, and ultimately you leave the trail below the level of the tracks. For now, however, you will be able to see more and more of the river (still the Minnesota) and get glimpses of the tracks.

By mile 2.8 you will have had several chances to see the river activity below (now the Mississippi) and possibly watched, listened, and felt as a few trains went by. You will also come upon the first of three kiosks set up at rest points along the trail. These mini-overlooks have a couple of benches and provide information about the historical and geological past of the region. The first kiosk discusses the confluence of the rivers below. If you look directly across the river you will also see the shoreline fronting Crosby Farm, another hiking area that is included in this book (see facing page). Pike Island is just downstream, with the Minnesota River entering from the left (east) side of that island.

There are two more informational kiosks, spaced about 0.3 mile apart, which explain more of the area's history, culture, and geology. The river, train tracks, and trail are just about 50 yards apart at this point. The surface of the trail is only about 15 feet above the river level.

As the trail approaches the northern terminus, the trees close in again, forming a corridor umbrella of box elders, ironwoods, maples, ashes, and lindens. The trees and honeysuckle understory in this section seemed especially alive with songbirds, and I experienced frequent sightings along this route.

The trail drops below the railroad grade and comes out just beyond a trestle overpass on MN 13 a couple of hundred yards from the St. Paul Yacht Club. There are vault toilets, an informational kiosk, and a small, paved parking lot at this end of the trail.

If I wanted to enjoy the river portion of this hike, I would drop my car at the Lilydale/Yacht Club end of the trail and walk along the river to the Mendota Heights section and back. This river-view section of the hike offers the most natural features and superb vistas. Besides, everything always looks different from the opposite direction.

NEARBY ACTIVITIES

There are segments of trails along the river farther north into Lilydale that can be hiked beyond the official length of the Big Rivers trail. Likewise, there are a few link-ups to other Dakota County trails beyond the southern terminus. If you drive over the bridge toward Minneapolis, you can drop down to either Fort Snelling State Park or Crosby Farm Park (and the adjoining trail to Hidden Falls) for even more extensions on these trails. Ultimately you can link to more than 72 miles of the Mississippi National River and Recreation Area.

CROSBY FARM PARK 3

IN BRIEF

Crosby Farm contains a hidden patch of history right at the confluence of the Mississippi and Minnesota rivers. Trails follow the river and wind through the bottomlands and marshes beneath the sheer bluffs near downtown St. Paul.

DESCRIPTION

There's a lot of history along the Mississippi River, some of it big and bold, like Fort Snelling, and some barely noticeable beyond the bluff line. Such is the case with Crosby Farm.

When Thomas Crosby and his wife, Emma, first came to this site on the Mississippi River in 1858, they found an area already bustling with activity. Fort Snelling, completed in 1825 to protect early settlers, loomed on the bluffs above Pike Island. Just downstream, a growing settlement founded by "Pig's Eye" Perrant would eventually become St. Paul. Crosby, an English immigrant, found 160 acres in the floodplain of the Mississippi River, just beyond the point where the Minnesota joins the Mississippi, and settled just downstream

- -

Directions ————————————————▶

From Ford Parkway, drive south on Cleveland to Mississippi River Boulevard, and turn left on Shepard Road; park entrances are on the right. The second exit is on the right after another 1.5 miles. From I-35 East in downtown St. Paul, take the Shepard Road exit west to Crosby Road and the eastern park entrance. For the western park entrance, go 1.5 miles past the eastern entrance to the marina sign. Turn left and follow the road past the marina to the entrance and Crosby Farm Museum. From MN 55, go north to MN 5, exit at Shepard Road, and follow the directions above.

KEY AT-A-GLANCE INFORMATION

LENGTH: 2.8 miles (side trails and cut-throughs add a mile or so more)

CONFIGURATION: Elongated figure eight with additional shortcuts and extensions up and down the river

DIFFICULTY: Flat bottomlands can be slippery when wet and muddy.

SCENERY: Classic Mississippi River bottomlands; extended and frequent views of the river and Pike Island

EXPOSURE: Mostly shaded, with morning sun along riverbank

TRAFFIC: Peaceful, with an undiscovered feeling about it

TRAIL SURFACE: Wide, paved walkway with one section of boardwalk

HIKING TIME: 1–2 hours

SEASON: Year-round; great for skiing or snowshoeing in winter

ACCESS: No fees

MAPS: Check at Nature Center or tinyurl.com/83ejfov

FACILITIES: Nature center, picnic area; no other development

SPECIAL COMMENTS: You literally drop down out of the Twin Cities and into an area that looks the same as it did when first farmed 150 years ago.

CONTACT: (651) 632-5111

GPS TRAILHEAD COORDINATES

Latitude   N93° 9.750'
Longitude   W44° 53.929'

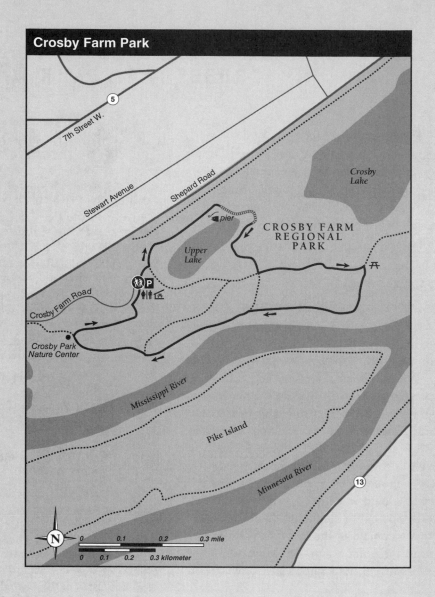

on the Mississippi from Fort Snelling. Today this narrow 2-mile-long floodplain is Crosby Farm Regional Park. The site of the old Crosby farm is at the southern end of the park. Trails run along the base of the bluff line, across marshy areas, and parallel to the river throughout this slice of river bottomland.

There are two entrances to this park, both off Shepard Road. This hike begins at the westernmost (or southern) entrance. It's the same entrance used for the marina.

Begin at the second parking lot beyond the museum; there the trail heads north through alders and willows to the south end of Upper Lake. Upper and Crosby lakes are nestled close to the base of the bluffs. Fed by the spring floods of the Mississippi, these two lakes are shallow and their banks are lined with marsh vegetation.

The trail forks at Upper Lake: one trail heads to the left and goes between the bluff and the lake, while the other goes right along the south edge of the marsh. This loop is an interpretive trail featuring two dozen stations with information on the flora and fauna of the area. For this hike, take the left fork and go around the lake, enjoying the wooden walkway at the northern third of the lake. If you take the right fork, you will soon come to the intersection with the left trail as it loops around Upper Lake. Otherwise the trail continues toward the river.

Some 40 yards farther, you'll come to an intersection with two other trails. This junction offers you three options. The trail to the left follows the eastern side of Crosby Lake and leads to the north entrance of the park. You can take this out-and-back for an extra mile of hiking. Gigantic cottonwood trees, some more than 6 feet in diameter, highlight this trail.

The trail to the right cuts through the center of the park. At the southern end you can either circle back along the river or continue on to the picnic shelter near the park entrance.

However, we'll continue on by going straight through the intersection and following the trail that leads to the river and then swings south (right), taking you down the riverbank and through the lowlands back to the far southern end of Crosby Park.

The trail follows the curve and contour of the banks of the Mississippi River. Huge cottonwood trees stand along the shoreline like sentinels guarding the river. There's not much understory here—it's all been swept away by repeated high waters in the spring. Most of the other trees throughout the area are ash and maple. Sometimes there's a tangle of downed trees and broken limbs, but mostly it's an open area with small plants doing their best to be tall on one season's growth.

Since a major flooding in the summer of 2000, this area is slowly regaining its understory litter. Still, some places have large areas of very fine sand stretching many, many yards back from the river. In the fall, the maple leaves on this barren but sandy forest floor give the area an almost surreal appearance, especially with low autumn sun cutting through the trees.

Occasionally, you will find trails leading off through the floodplain or continuing along the river as the main trail turns inward. These all end up connecting to the main loop—they've been carved out of the understory by years of creative bushwhacking.

The trail continues along the river for the full length of the park. You can look to the south (out across the river) and practically throw a stone onto Pike Island. Imagine the activity in this area 150 years ago. Today, it's a quiet, casual park hidden below the banks of the river that created it. It's like a mini Fort Snelling Park, only less crowded.

The trail cuts back into the bottomlands, where it intersects with the trail that bisects the park parallel to the river (the second trail choice you had back at

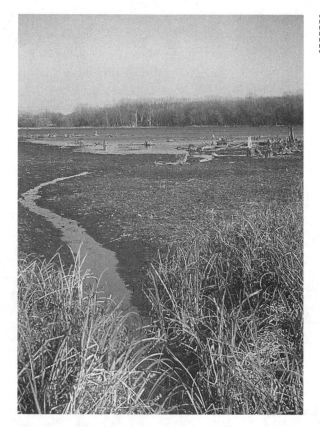

Crosby Lake offers a classic example of Mississippi River bottomlands.

the covered shelter). Take a left at the intersection to head to the picnic area or stay to the right to reconnect with the Upper Lake Trail, at which point you can take a left and backtrack a short distance to return to the trailhead.

NEARBY ACTIVITIES

If you want, you can connect to the Hidden Falls hike. Hidden Falls is a small waterfall cut high into the bluffs of the Mississippi River, above the dam and not too far north of where the creek from Minnehaha Falls empties into the river. The falls are not visible from above or below, but a short trail leads there from either direction. The flowage is infrequent and sparse, but the little forested cove in which it's nestled offers some solitude along the busy river boulevard. Hidden Falls is accessible from the river trail leading out of Crosby Farm. To reach it from Crosby Farm, continue along the paved trail outside the park entrance and past the marina. There is a gate through which you can walk to connect with a paved corridor to Hidden Falls—a 1.5-mile one-way hike. Taking this optional out-and-back will give you another 3 miles of hiking.

LAKE ELMO PARK RESERVE,
Eagle Point Lake

 4

IN BRIEF

Mostly wetlands and forests, Lake Elmo Park features two main lakes, open meadows, and more types and numbers of evergreens than most area parks. This trail keeps the lake in sight for most of its length while still taking in some of the park's rolling meadows.

DESCRIPTION

Access Eagle Point Lake from the central trailhead in the park's first parking lot.

Leaving the marsh grasses and cattails behind, take Trail 19 uphill into the stand of upland oaks and maples. One of the first things that stood out to me about this park was the number of evergreens—spruce, cedar, and white pine—that grow in clusters throughout the entire area. You are heading south, so stay on this trail and continue past the intersection with Trail 17 on your left. You want to stay on Trail 19 through these uplands and around the south end of the lake. You will find more oaks, maples, and ashes growing as little wooded islands in the meadows. Most of the meadows are bordered by rows of trees—primarily pines.

Located close to a major freeway (I-694), this park has a constant buzz from that traffic. Open meadows are particularly susceptible to such ambient noise, as are any of the smaller wooded areas that have lost their sound-buffering leaves late in the season. Fortunately, this is the only section of the hike where I

Directions

From Minneapolis or St. Paul, drive east on I-94 to CR 19 (Exit 251). Go north on CR 19 for 1 mile to park entrance. Follow road into park to first parking lot on left; go to end of parking lot for main trailhead.

---

i KEY AT-A-GLANCE INFORMATION

LENGTH: 3.7 miles

CONFIGURATION: Irregular circle following elevation around the lake

DIFFICULTY: Easy throughout, with a couple of minor elevation changes

SCENERY: A patchwork of meadows surrounding a marsh grass–lined pond; a sunny summer day is the best time for this very picturesque park.

EXPOSURE: Mostly full sun, except for wooded area around trailhead

TRAFFIC: Moderately busy in summer and fall

TRAIL SURFACE: Medium-wide, mowed grassy lanes

HIKING TIME: 1.5–2 hours

SEASON: Year-round; very wide ski/skate trail in winter

ACCESS: $5 daily; $25 annual; reciprocity with Carver and Anoka County parks

MAPS: Available at park or at www.co.washington.mn.us/parks

FACILITIES: Campground with electricity, restrooms, showers, picnic area, playground, swimming at Lake Elmo

SPECIAL COMMENTS: Lake Elmo is a popular boating/fishing lake.

CONTACT: (651) 430-8370

GPS TRAILHEAD COORDINATES

Latitude   N92° 54.294'

Longitude   W44° 58.531'

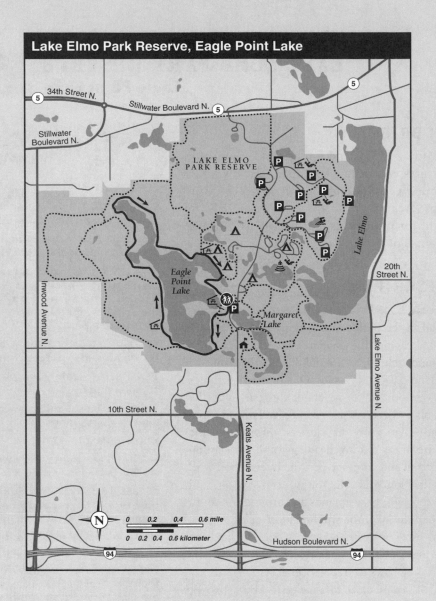

found the traffic hum even noticeable. Mature paper birches, maples, cotton-woods, and a few fine-needled white pines grow throughout this section.

Continue around toward the western edge of the lake, where hardwoods give way to open grasslands characteristic of the oak prairie. It is hilly country sprinkled with wildflowers and edged with spruce. Some of these trails double as horse and cross-country skiing trails. This trail has a gravelly surface—soft, but noisy.

Eventually you will come to the Trail 30 junction. It cuts to the left away from the lake. Ignore any signs, and stay to the right to continue around the lake. Eagle Point Lake is shallow, with many stretches of shoreline thick with marsh grass. The entire lake covers 143 acres and, because it is so shallow, it does not support fishing.

The trail continues through an older growth of hardwoods and gains elevation. Soon it reaches a high point overlooking the lake. A large ski shelter with two picnic tables sits on a knoll overlooking Eagle Point. The trail rises another 20 feet to an area of gently rolling fields bursting with goldenrod in the fall. This expanse is bordered on the left by red oaks. The trail follows the contours of the field in gradual, but even, 10-foot changes in elevation—the hills resemble a series of swells on the ocean.

Arriving at the intersection of Trail 29, look to the west to see more pockets of oaks scattered across the prairie. The open nature of this park, coupled with the high number of evergreens, contributes to its charm. Continue past the intersection, and in another 150 yards you get a good view of the northwest end of Eagle Point Lake.

White-tailed deer abound in the park, evidenced by numerous deer tracks on the trail and the lanes of tracks that crisscross the trail. The intersection of Trail 28 is easy to spot because of a prominent landmark rising tall out of the grass: an old windmill from a former homestead. Many of the surrounding meadows are lined in evergreens—a subtle reminder that this land was once farmed. Crops grew in the meadows, and the lines of evergreens were planted as windbreaks.

You'll encounter Trail 16 next, a short punch through the thick, wooded area to the right. It appears to lead through a boggy area and across a narrow drainage flowing out of the north end of Eagle Point. If you take this spur it will save you 0.6 mile of walking around another pond and a boggy area at the northernmost end of Eagle Point.

However, if you go the extra distance, you'll find that it's easy walking. Continue past this shortcut to see more of the pond on the right. The trail follows the pond's oblong shape and loops around its northern end. This area struck me as potentially being very picturesque in the spring. The trail skirts the marshy area to the right before circling back around the top of the loop. You'll come across more red oaks here, too.

Located at this loop is a knoll of oaks to your left. Check out the ruins of a foundation for some sort of building or dock. At this point on the trail you have reached the far end of the 3.7-mile loop. A few paces down the trail and 300 yards to the left (beyond the field) is a private residence. Turn around and catch the lovely vista down the entire length of the pond and Eagle Point Lake beyond. From this vantage point the pond appears to be an elongated S shape. You can see the narrow band of land between Eagle Point and the pond, as well as the shortcut Trail 16.

You are near what appears to be the highest point in the park, at least from this vantage point. Open fields spread to the east in long rectangles bordered by more evergreens. This edge of the lake has a lot of deadfall and thick, tangled underbrush. The habitat looks perfect for raccoons, foxes, and other critters. Deer tracks abound here as well. Continue down the trail, passing by the marker for Trail 15 on your right, the other end of the 0.6-mile shortcut.

The trail turns east, flanked by cottonwoods, dogwoods on the right, and what might have been a wheat field or other planting on the left. A bit farther on you'll come upon a small pond on your left and the intersection with Trail 21. Here you'll see a cluster of pin oaks and cedars. Trail 21 leads left to the campground and connects with other loops. Instead, turn right and continue down a short but steep pathway, over a drainage area, and past the intersection with Trail 14, which leads back to the campground (and links up with another trail to the parking lot). If you look over your left shoulder you can catch a glimpse of Lake Elmo.

The last segment of the trail follows along a ridge and is now paralleling the park road about 50 yards through the trees to the left. Any of the next spurs will take you to the main park road and parking area beyond the trailhead.

NEARBY ACTIVITIES

Need more trails? There are several minor loops across the road. Trails 1 and 2 will take you to the south end of Lake Elmo.

SOUTH ST. PAUL RIVERFRONT TRAIL 5

IN BRIEF

This passive trail parallels the Mighty Mississippi with opportunities to see river and railroad commerce in action while enjoying sweeping views along the river and across to the wooded shoreline.

DESCRIPTION

If you are into trains, barges, and big, slow-flowing rivers, then this is the trail for you. There's not a lot of glamour in this paved path that follows the shoreline of the Mississippi as it flows past downtown St. Paul. The east bank is tree lined and gives the illusion that expansive forests lie beyond the waters. Not so the west bank. This is the industrial side of this section of the river. The trail runs immediately parallel to an extensive railroad yard with multiple tracks, idling locomotives, and a repository of boxcars. It's not a wooded wonderland, but it is a representation of the commercial lifeblood of this magnificent river. If you don't enjoy the natural scenery, you can't help but appreciate the commerce created on the river.

Directions ─────────────────➤

From I-94 in downtown St. Paul, go south on US 52 (Exit 242) about 2 miles to Concord Street (CR 156). Follow Concord Street south about 1.25 miles to Simon's Ravine Park on right (just beyond pedestrian bridge over Concord). The DNR access ramp and southern trailhead are west off of Concord onto Armour Avenue (0.75 mile north of I-494). Take a right on Hardman Avenue, and go south 0.5 mile to Verderosa Avenue. Take a left, and follow back south under I-494 to the ramp immediately on the left.

KEY AT-A-GLANCE INFORMATION

LENGTH: 4 miles

CONFIGURATION: Point to point (with out-and-back option)

DIFFICULTY: Mostly level trail with a few short, gradual inclines

SCENERY: A few short sections of scattered vegetation along mostly open embankment/levee above Mississippi River in urban-industrial setting with broad vistas along and across the river

EXPOSURE: Fully exposed throughout entire trail

TRAFFIC: Mostly bike traffic with frequent hiking use

TRAIL SURFACE: 8-foot-wide paved surface throughout

HIKING TIME: 1.5 hours

SEASON: Year-round

ACCESS: No fee for hiking

MAPS: Online at southstpaul.org

FACILITIES: Restrooms and drinking fountain at Simon's Raven Park entrance

SPECIAL COMMENTS: This trail parallels railroad tracks for much of its length; broad vistas along and across the Mississippi River on one side are coupled by the railroad corridor behind commercial sites along the other side of the river.

CONTACT: (651) 306-3690

GPS TRAILHEAD COORDINATES

Latitude   N93° 3.247'

Longitude   W44° 54.744'

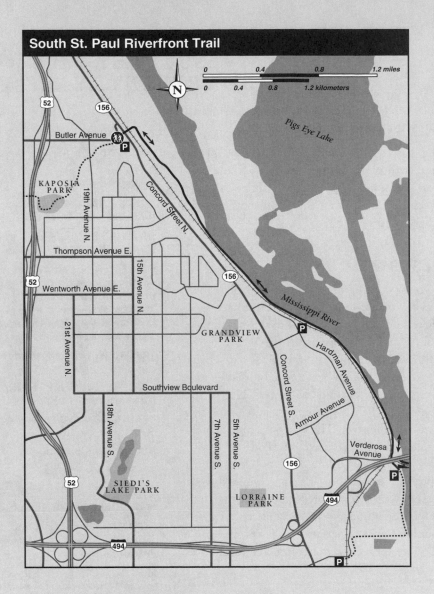

South St. Paul Riverfront Trail

With that in mind, this trail is a good example of South St. Paul's efforts to provide modern, clean, and well-laid-out parks and waysides. This trail starts at Simon's Ravine, about a mile from the heart of downtown. It begins at a junction of two trails: the riverfront trail I recommend, and the Simon's Ravine Trail that leads up through the ravine into Kaposia Park and links up to another trail covered in this book—the Thompson Park trail (see page 37). Here again, extensive trails have been routed through natural corridors in the heart of a major metropolitan city. Gotta love it!

From the Simon's Ravine Trailhead parking lot, head right and up and around the pedestrian/bike overpass bridge. This brings you to a huge, long grassy field above the river. A trail runs along the perimeter of this area for brisk workouts or short, looped jaunts. Continue down the path to an intersection at the north end of the off-leash-dog compound ahead. The trail skirts the western border of this area, but take the left and head toward the river. There you will come to a T. To the left is the loop around the huge lawn. You want to go right and head down along the river. This section follows the river edge of the expansive open grassy area, and then swings right to connect with the main trail that has now continued on past the dog area.

The main trail is now heading south high above the river atop the levee that secures the embankment on this side of the channel. You can reach out and almost touch the boxcars just beyond the fence on your right. A better option would be to enjoy the benches on the left that offer a view down to and across the river.

There are several places along the route where vegetation and lowland trees block the view of the river. These are short segments, and more often than not the route offers unobstructed views downstream. Barge traffic and the lazy current provide a constant visual flow as you walk along.

Several hundred yards down a long, exposed straightaway, the trail slopes upward as it comes to a different section of the levee. A picnic table on a gravel turnout sits at the crest of the slope. This might be a good place to stop and watch people fish along the bank or from a scattering of small fishing boats that tend to converge here.

It should be noted that there are no amenities along this trail, and the exposed, paved path laid out on a stone levee can get unbearably hot during the summer. There is water at the Simon's Ravine Trailhead, so make sure you have plenty of filled water bottles and a sun hat.

About a mile before you cross under the I-494 bridge, a broad, spiraling stairway up and over the railroad tracks on the right leads to a parking area on Grand Avenue. Just a few blocks off of Concord Street, this parking area could serve as a car-drop point if you wanted to cut this trip about 1.5 miles short of its southern terminus.

Just beyond the ramp is a 2-mile marker that I believe designates the distance from the official southern end of the riverfront hike—about 1.5 miles beyond where I suggest ending.

The trail slopes back down, off the higher levee as it were, as it continues past a cluster of vegetation on the river side of the trail. Wildflower Levee Park is about 0.5 mile beyond the stairway overpass and features several picnic tables overlooking the Mississippi. From here the trail skirts a backwater area on the left as a long concrete wall hugs the right side of the trail for several hundred yards. Looking down the trail, you will get your first clear glimpse of the elevated spans carrying the multiple lanes of I-494 still 0.5 mile away.

Just after crossing under the highway you'll notice a newer, smoother (probably patched) section of the already smoothly paved trail. This hike ends at the Department of Natural Resources (DNR) boat ramp. There is ample parking down below the trail and a few benches placed along the open riverbank beyond the

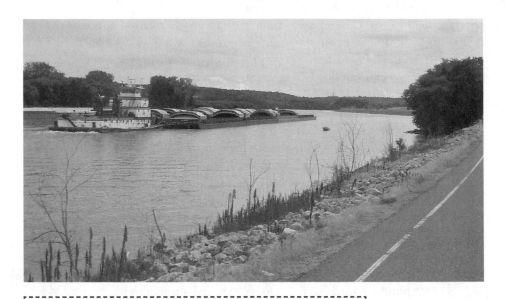

Barge traffic is part of the commerce along the South St. Paul trail corridor.

ramp. You could park here and do an out-and-back to the north end, or take the remaining 1.5 miles of trail to the official southern end.

From the DNR ramp south, the trail drops down into a stand of trees bounded on the right by a gravel pit work area. Just before its southern end, the trail crosses the railroad tracks and fuses into city streets and residential bike lanes. There is a small parking lot behind a warehouse (signage reads REGIONAL TRAIL PARKING).

If you are still eager for additional hiking but need to feel more enclosed in greenery, head back to the trailhead and take a trip up through Simon's Ravine. As soon as you travel up the draw, there is a fork in the trail. It is a short spur that reconnects with the main trail after crossing a short footbridge. It winds up through the woods to Kaposia Park (and a disc-golf complex) before crossing the highway and continuing into the southeast section of Thompson County Park, where its trail system winds through hilly, tree-covered terrain.

While it's not the most scenic nor the prettiest trail in this guide, the South St. Paul Riverfront Trail does offer a sense of river life and an imaginative feel of what it was like living along a river of such magnitude. A lot of history has flowed along this river; this trail may enable you to think about those days as you stroll along its banks.

NEARBY ACTIVITIES

The trail is located just south of downtown St. Paul and within blocks of a diverse Mexican neighborhood with Hispanic shops and eateries over a several-block area. The trailhead links up with a short hike up a wooded ravine that eventually leads to a southern access point to the Thompson County Park trail to the west.

THOMPSON COUNTY PARK,
Thompson Trail

6

IN BRIEF

This is a small neighborhood park with a modest lake and pleasant oak stands to hike through. The trail is short but has a more remote flavor once you get back into the hilly woods.

DESCRIPTION

The Thompson County hiking trail cuts several paths through this tiny chunk of big woods tucked in between the freeway and houses on St. Paul's south side. Entering the park, the impression is one of a country wayside next to a very small lake. For the most part, that's exactly right.

The hiking trail begins at the parking lot and follows the paved pathway around the front of the information center. The path heads down to the small, pondlike body of water called Thompson Lake. Turn right at the intersection and follow the path, which is paved around the developed half of the lake. Just after a footbridge over the creek at the northern end of the lake, the path turns into a crushed-gravel path about 5 feet wide. The path continues around the lake and is flanked by sumacs on the shore side and a buffer zone of grasses between the park and the adjoining neighborhood on the right.

Although very small (the entire park is only 57 acres), the lake was bustling with waterfowl activity the day I was there. Mallards, songbirds (mostly warblers), and even

Directions

Drive north on US 52 (Lafayette Freeway) to Butler Avenue. Turn left and drive to Stassen Lane. Turn left into the park, and stop at the first parking lot on the right.

KEY AT-A-GLANCE INFORMATION

LENGTH: 1.4 miles

CONFIGURATION: Figure eight

DIFFICULTY: Easy; rolling pathway with some steep inclines

SCENERY: Pleasantly woodsy with rolling hills

EXPOSURE: Lake is sunny, but rest of hike is shaded

TRAFFIC: Neighborhood park; moderate usage

TRAIL SURFACE: Trail around developed side of lake is paved; the rest is hard pack.

HIKING TIME: 1 hour

SEASON: Year-round; busy in winter due to lighted ski trails

ACCESS: No fees

MAPS: Available from Dakota County or at tinyurl.com/thompsontrail

FACILITIES: Picnic pavilion, restrooms, playground, telephone

SPECIAL COMMENTS: Corridor trails lead off from the 1-mile looped trail: the North Urban Regional Trail connects with the south-end trail in the park, and the Mississippi River Regional Trail heads east, across US 52, through Kaposia Park and comes out by the river at Simon's Ravine Park and the trailhead for the South St. Paul Riverfront Trail.

CONTACT: (651) 437-3191

GPS TRAILHEAD COORDINATES

Latitude	N93° 4.191'
Longitude	W44° 54.692'

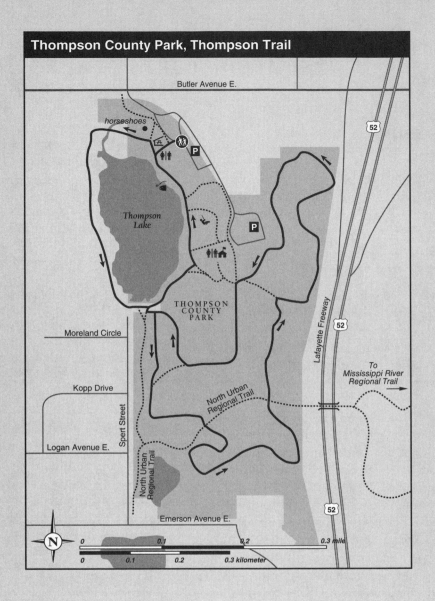

horseshoes

Thompson Lake

THOMPSON COUNTY PARK

Butler Avenue E.

Moreland Circle

Kopp Drive

Logan Avenue E.

Spert Street

North Urban Regional Trail

North Urban Regional Trail

Lafayette Freeway

To Mississippi River Regional Trail

Emerson Avenue E.

52

52

52

N

| 0 | 0.1 | 0.2 | 0.3 mile |
| 0 | 0.1 | 0.2 | 0.3 kilometer |

an egret took their places along the little nicks in the otherwise even shoreline of the oval lake.

The trail continues south into woods and patchy open areas. At the bottom of this lake loop, you'll see a trail heading right, a continuation of the gravel trail. The first turn to the right is a continuation of the paved trail out of the park. Stay on the main route, and take the second grass trail that angles up a modest grassy knoll and heads into the island of trees ahead.

In this section you have a number of options to create hikes of varying lengths. For our hike, we'll follow the perimeter of this trail system to create a

1-mile loop. Continue down the trail and ignore the path heading off to your left—this will be where you return in a little while. Shortly after this intersection you'll come to a fork. The path to the left goes about 0.2 mile and intersects with the larger loop trail. Stay to the right, however, and follow the loop along the southern half of the park.

This southern part of the park, like the rest of the wooded area, features abundant oaks and maples. Its topography and tree cover are typical of this area before development leveled off or filled in the natural wooded areas. The hilliness is reminiscent of glacial deposited kames and kettle areas nearby. In fact, it is part of the St. Croix glacial moraine.

The loop cuts across the bottom third of the park and then meets and parallels the park's eastern boundary alongside US 52. The trail returns north and in 90 yards intersects with the trail that leads back to the fork you passed earlier. The trail soon approaches another intersection, that of the spur that leads out of the park toward the river and other trails to the east. You can also take a short jaunt down the left path to reach one of the highest points in the park. Continue on the main trail, heading north to enjoy another 0.5-mile loop that encircles the northeastern end of the park.

More oaks and upland understory are common throughout this area. The trail does move away from the freeway slightly before it circles around to come out at the small parking lot at the end of the park entrance road. Follow the trail to the left, and it will take you to the southern end of the lake. Take another right and follow the lakeshore back to the starting point at the parking lot.

NEARBY ACTIVITIES

The Mississippi River lies a few miles to the east. A segment of the Mississippi River Regional Trail can be accessed for a short hike along the river by turning right (east) on Butler Avenue after exiting the park and crossing Concord Street (CR 156) to the river. There are turnouts along the roadway and a few parking areas along the trail.

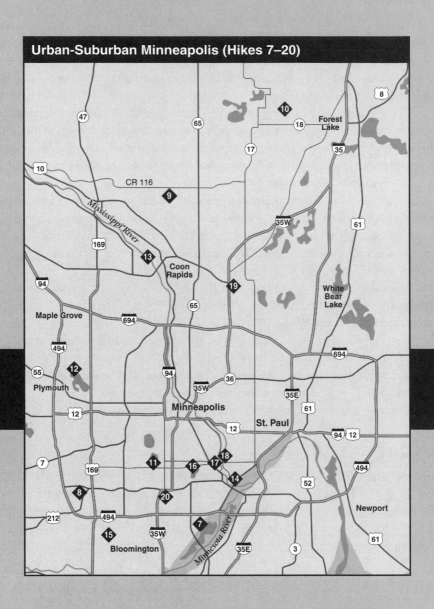

Urban-Suburban Minneapolis (Hikes 7–20)

URBAN-SUBURBAN
MINNEAPOLIS

7 BASS PONDS TRAIL,
Long Meadow Lake

KEY AT-A-GLANCE INFORMATION

LENGTH: 3 miles (0.5-mile interpretive loop and 1.25-mile out-and-back)

CONFIGURATION: Balloon

DIFFICULTY: Easy, mostly level river-bottom trails with few rises; may be slippery during spring and summer

SCENERY: Wide vistas over a large marshy/open-water lake; beautiful with early morning or evening sun

EXPOSURE: Shaded along banks, sunny in meadow and marsh areas

TRAFFIC: Single path along lake is less crowded than pond area; during the school year, the ponds are popular field classrooms for area schools.

TRAIL SURFACE: Packed turf/earth

HIKING TIME: 45–60 minutes for pond; 30 minutes to Old Cedar Avenue

SEASON: Year-round; use snowshoes and skis during winter

ACCESS: No fees

MAPS: Available at Refuge Headquarters off of I-494 and 34th Avenue, and at Bass Ponds Environmental Study Area kiosk

FACILITIES: Parking, kiosk

SPECIAL COMMENTS: The opportunity to connect with the Old Cedar Avenue trail is a bonus.

CONTACT: (952) 854-5900

GPS TRAILHEAD COORDINATES

Latitude   N93° 14.129'

Longitude   W44° 50.865'

IN BRIEF

The Minnesota Valley National Wildlife Refuge is only 10 miles from downtown Minneapolis. That and its 34 miles of river bottoms teeming with wildlife and natural amenities make it one of only four urban wildlife refuges in the United States. In my book, it's one of the very best places to hike in the Twin Cities. Urban wildlife- and bird-watchers should put this on the top of their list of premier viewing areas near Minneapolis and St. Paul.

DESCRIPTION

The Bass Ponds are fun to explore along their own 0.5-mile hiking trail, and because it's another 1.25 miles down to the Old Cedar Bridge Trail (and another 1.25 miles back), I've decided to describe these as two distinct trails. The best way to enjoy these trails may be to go out and hike to the other end of the trail and then retrace your steps back to the initial trailhead—rehiking the entire path and seeing things from the other direction.

A second option would be to put a shuttle vehicle at the opposite end of this trail so you don't have to retrace your route.

The vehicle gate to the Bass Ponds is always locked. Those with disabilities can get a key beforehand at the refuge visitor center.

Directions ——————————➤

Entrance is located about 2 miles west of the Minnesota Valley National Wildlife Refuge Visitor Center. Take I-494 to the 24th Avenue exit; turn south past the Mall of America, and turn left (east) on East 86th Street. Follow 86th for about a block. As the road swings to the right, there is a sign on the driveway to the left that leads to a parking lot at the gated entrance to the Bass Ponds.

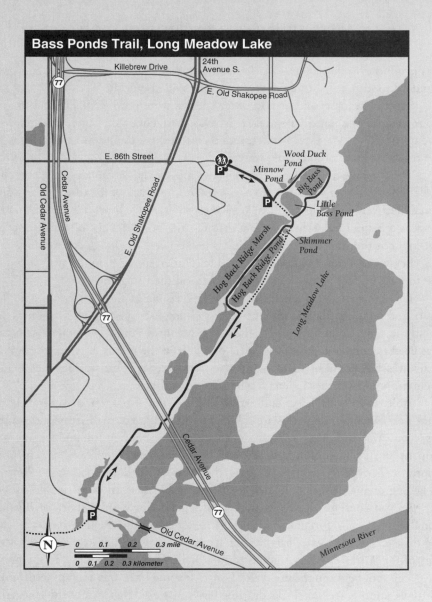

Bass Ponds Trail, Long Meadow Lake

Killebrew Drive
24th Avenue S.
E. Old Shakopee Road
77
E. 86th Street
Wood Duck Pond
Minnow Pond
Big Bass Pond
Little Bass Pond
Skimmer Pond
Hog Back Ridge Marsh
Hog Back Ridge Pond
Cedar Avenue
Old Cedar Avenue
E. Old Shakopee Road
Long Meadow Lake
77
Cedar Avenue
77
Old Cedar Avenue
Minnesota River
N
0   0.1   0.2   0.3 mile
0   0.1   0.2   0.3 kilometer

The roadway from the parking lot winds down into the lowlands. There, the river flats provide a nice transition from the suburban buzz of the freeway and the residential neighborhood above.

Once you reach the bottom, you can obtain details about the area's historic and natural amenities from the information kiosk. Originally used by state officials as bass-rearing ponds back in the 1920s, this area was in operation for more than 30 years. A spring-fed creek along the bottomlands provided the perfect aquatic conditions to create rearing ponds for more than 2.5 million largemouth bass. New breeding ponds were added in 1938, at which time experiments to produce a cross between a muskie and a northern pike were conducted. A hybrid was produced—one that grew so fast it began cannibalizing its own whenever its standard food supply of minnows was not provided quickly.

Sunfish, crappie, and myriad other species were produced here and used to stock lakes in the immediate area as well as throughout the state of Minnesota. Today the ponds are used as interpretive education sites and as resting areas for the region's flocks of migrating waterfowl.

The 0.5-mile trail network forms a big loop around the ponds in the complex. Called the Caretaker's Walk, it offers information on each of the various-size ponds that collectively make up the Bass Ponds. (An interpretive brochure available at the kiosk is a helpful tool when walking through the ponds.) This loop will also put you right at the start of the 1.25-mile trail southwest to Old Cedar Avenue.

Begin at the information kiosk and take a left along the interpretive trail to the first of 11 sites along the trail (as shown on the refuge map).

Remnants of the original operation are visible at the first two stops. The stairs and decaying foundation of the first clubhouse can be seen as soon as you begin the trail. Continuing on, to the left is Minnow Pond. The pillbox structure was used to control the flow and level of water in the ponds. Upstream from this pond was the home of the area's native brook trout. Cold springwater helped them grow 6–10 inches in length while living in the creek.

Walk another 100 feet and arrive at the Wood Duck Pond. Several wood-duck nests were put up in this area. The scientific name of such areas is green tree reservoir. Water collects in these depressions long enough for puddle ducks to stop by during migration and feed on seeds and plants on the bottom. Once migration is over and summer follows, these reservoirs dry up, allowing the trees to keep growing. If they remained full of water, many of the trees would drown.

As you continue down the trail, you begin following the shore of Big Bass Pond on your right. Imagine a crew of laborers digging this pond by hand and carting off excess dirt in wheelbarrows. That's how this was built in the late 1930s as part of the Works Progress Administration. Black crappie were raised in the pond.

The spot between the pond and Long Meadow Lake was a jumping-off point for duck hunters seeking flocks of game birds that used this area of the lake. Also, there was a commercial fishery where fishermen used to drop gill nets through cuts in the ice to catch carp for a cannery.

Heading southwest, the trail crosses a bridge over the creek from Minnow Pond and continues past Little Bass Pond's southern bank. Because willow trees root fast and love lots of water and wet soil, they were planted along these ponds so their roots could be used to secure the ponds' embankments.

Just past this pond is the intersection with a main trail that can take you back to the information kiosk. This is also the trailhead for the 1.25-mile out-and-back trail down to the Old Cedar Avenue Bridge. The next 0.25 mile continues along the ponds. In the winter, the large pond, called Hog Back Ridge Pond, doesn't always freeze over. Scores of Canada geese and various winter ducks can be seen here.

The trail along Long Meadow Lake continues for about 1 mile and traces the

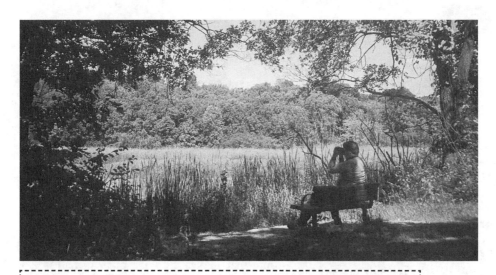

The author pauses for some bird-watching on a bench along the Old Cedar Avenue Trail.

edge of the lake. Towering cottonwoods and other lowland trees flank the banks for most of its length. This is an incredible birding area. In fact, the entire Minnesota Valley is one of the best corridors in the state for viewing all sorts of birds, both residents and transient migrators. Great blue herons, egrets, puddle ducks, swamp sparrows, and redwing and yellow-headed blackbirds are among hundreds of bird species that can be seen along Long Meadow Lake's shoreline. Be sure to bring your spotting scope or binoculars.

Once you pass under MN 77 (Cedar Avenue), you enter marshlands and eventually come upon a few smaller ponds on each side of the road. The terminus of Bass Ponds Trail is at Old Cedar Avenue. The trail comes out across from the parking lot, the trailhead for the Cedar Trail and the old steel-frame bridge that once carried traffic south along Old Cedar Avenue. The bridge is now closed to all traffic.

At this point you have several choices: continue on the Old Cedar Avenue trail network; retrace your steps back to the Bass Ponds area; continue along Long Meadow Lake Trail another couple of miles to its western terminus at I-35 West; or get in the shuttle car you placed here before you started your trip. Pick a nice, sunny Minnesota day for your hike, and you may have a hard time deciding what to do next.

NEARBY ACTIVITIES

The trail-system options for the Minnesota Valley National Wildlife Refuge are the first activities that come to mind. At least four other trail systems feed off this trail at the southern terminus and beyond. For a totally different walking experience, try hiking the four levels of the great Mall of America just up the road (its doors open early to allow walkers access to the corridor levels).

8 BRYANT LAKE

KEY AT-A-GLANCE INFORMATION

LENGTH: 1.3 miles

CONFIGURATION: A very irregular, amoebalike balloon

DIFFICULTY: Undulating, with some slippery sections

SCENERY: Oak savanna at higher elevations with developing topography from steep slopes

EXPOSURE: Mostly full sun; marshy area in shade

TRAFFIC: Some along the marshy interior—deer take refuge here

TRAIL SURFACE: Paved walkways

HIKING TIME: 45–60 minutes

SEASON: Spring–fall

ACCESS: No fees

MAPS: Available at park headquarters or at threeriversparks.org

FACILITIES: Fully developed with picnic area, visitor center, restrooms, water

SPECIAL COMMENTS: Plenty of parking—a nice short hike for busy people

CONTACT: (763) 694-7764

GPS TRAILHEAD COORDINATES

Latitude   N93° 25.174'

Longitude   W44° 53.059'

IN BRIEF

Noted for its steep, rolling hills, the park's trail network enables hikers to combine a walking workout with glimpses of nature's handiwork preserved in a bustling urban setting.

DESCRIPTION

Surrounded by freeways, townhouses, and more highways, the Bryant Lake Trail is a modest route that makes the most of this small urban park. By capitalizing on every twist and turn within the park, the trail serves two purposes: one as a vigorous workout/power-walking loop; the other as a chance to relax and enjoy terrain and trees more common to rural parks. By combining both walking environments, you'll find that Bryant Lake offers a full-featured, albeit short, hike through the woods and marshy areas of the park's southeastern half.

Head down to the beach area, and start the hike along the paved trail that heads off into the woods beyond the canoe-rental building. This southeastern section of the park is in a much less developed area with a dense growth of native trees and other vegetation and hilly terrain bordering Medicine Lake.

As you climb the hill, the paved trail winds north past a cluster of picnic tables. Continuing on about 100 yards, you'll see a park road paralleling the trail and a parking lot beyond. The trail has a short spur that

---

Directions

Head west on Crosstown 62 to the intersection with US 212. Take US 212 west about 0.7 mile to Shady Oak Road/CR 61. Turn north/right, and go 0.3 mile to Rowland Road. Turn left and go about one block; then turn left into the park at the sign.

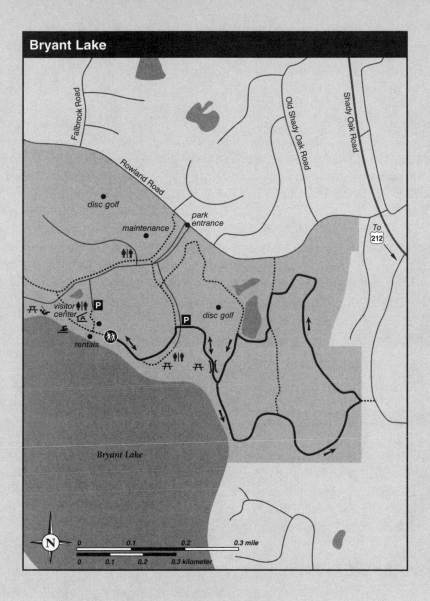

directs you across the road and then connects up with a continuation of the paved trail back down into the woods beyond the parking lot.

The steep, rolling hills are considered the most striking feature of the park. At the highest point in the park you will be almost 150 feet above the lake. Some of the slopes are quite steep. Between these extremely steep sides are valleylike chutes, called swales, that vary in width and all lead back down to the lake. The hills on this trail enable one to launch a power hike along the slopes.

The trail drops down toward the lake, bending to the right as it descends from the parking lot. As the trail levels off near the lake, it crosses a small footbridge over a creek. A grassy trail just before this bridge heads back to the right, along the lake back to the picnic area you passed earlier. The paved trail then swings inland along the southern edge of the marshland. The wooded areas are dominated by mature oaks and maples. Lower down the slopes toward the lake, the trees and understory are typical of floodplain flora found throughout this region, such as cottonwoods and ashes. This is in sharp contrast to the savannalike burr oaks, hawthorns, and red cedars found higher up in the central and western part of the park.

Just beyond the footbridge, a grassy path heads back from the lake and into the heart of the wooded area. Later, you will return via this trail from the other side of the loop.

The trail continues following the lake, then curves northward, before curving toward the lake again. At the top of curve the trail intersects another trail on the left. This is in a clearing with a maintenance building to the right of a gravel road. The trail goes into the woods to the north. It too is one of the options for a return back to the paved loop from the top of the grassy loop. You could take this left and cut about 0.4 mile off your hike. Don't! Stay on the paved trail as it loops around to the eastern boundary of the park.

Be on the lookout for deer. At dusk in October I witnessed four deer entering this wild area from the backyards of the nearby houses.

Once you reach the eastern edge of the park, the paved trail continues out of the park. Just before the paved trail reaches the street, take a left onto the grassy path and head back into the woods. You'll enjoy more dense foliage as you swing around the northern section of this trail. At the first of two intersecting trails, the trail heads back down to the maintenance building you passed earlier. Take it to the left and then take the next right that puts you back on the northern section heading west. A bit farther another trail heads south (left) again. Take it and head back down the trail, where you'll come out onto the paved trail just east of the footbridge. A right onto the paved trail leads you back to the start.

NEARBY ACTIVITIES

For such a small park, its amenities are impressive. The park has a modern visitor center, boat launch, and fishing pier. A trail leads out of the northwest end of the park and connects with trails from Eden Prairie and Minnetonka.

BUNKER HILLS REGIONAL PARK 9

IN BRIEF

A network of trails winds through these prairie and oak savanna hills, offering a large loop with spur trails to provide additional routes or shortcuts. The stands of oaks are impressive.

DESCRIPTION

This part of Anoka County is made up of sandy soil—so sandy that early attempts at farming failed. The county's Parks and Recreation Department created Bunker Hills in 1963 and since then has created a full-service regional park. Like everything else in this regional park, the 7.4 miles of 8-foot-wide, asphalt-covered hiking trails are well groomed, well maintained, and nicely laid out as part of an overall development plan that appears well organized and administrated.

This hike loops around the outer edge of the park's varied amenities and links up with trails that lead either out and back to specific areas, such as the horse stables, or that enable hikers to make numerous shortcuts to points within the loop. Because of the sandy soil, the predominant trees in this park are the mighty oaks. Sometimes pure stands of gnarly, stately oaks provide corridors through which hikers can enjoy the serpentine trail that winds, dips, and climbs ever so gently over the slightly hilly topography. Other stretches of the trail cut through fields of prairie grasses offering vistas across the park.

Directions _____→

Take I-35 West north to US 10 in Mounds View. Turn left (west) on US 10 (Exit 30) and go 2.5 miles to MN 65. Turn right (north) on MN 65 and go 4.2 miles to MN 242; then drive west on MN 242/CR 14 for 2.5 miles to the park entrance at Foley Boulevard.

KEY AT-A-GLANCE INFORMATION

LENGTH: 2.5 miles

CONFIGURATION: Irregular loop

DIFFICULTY: Easy

SCENERY: Groves of oak trees in a landscaped park setting with views of open fields and various developments in the park

EXPOSURE: Stretches of sun and shade intermittent throughout the hike

TRAFFIC: Multiuse trails popular with bicyclists and hikers

TRAIL SURFACE: Paved throughout

HIKING TIME: 1.5 hours

SEASON: Year-round

ACCESS: $5 daily parking fee per vehicle

MAPS: At Visitor Contact Station, activities center, or online at anokacountyparks.com

FACILITIES: Nearby park facilities include restrooms, water, interpretive center, picnic area, water park, campgrounds, and golf course

SPECIAL COMMENTS: This short, pleasant trail through a well-thought-out, full-service regional park includes many activities to enjoy in addition to hiking.

CONTACT: (763) 757-3920

GPS TRAILHEAD COORDINATES

Latitude   N93° 16.863'

Longitude   W45° 12.352'

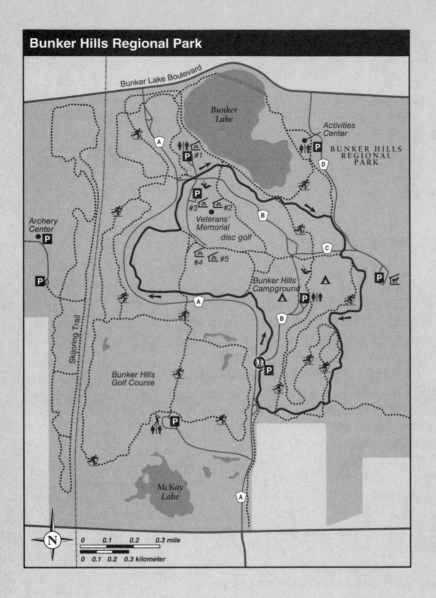

The trail also brings hikers close to some of the recreational opportunities of this diverse park. Bunker Hills is probably best known for Bunker Beach and the incredible wave pool, Minnesota's only artificial surf–generating water park. The trail also links up with the road through both campgrounds, the rustic site, and the RV camping area.

This hike actually starts just outside the road to the campgrounds at a small parking lot right on the trail system. Almost immediately, the trail leads through a solid stand of mostly burr oaks mixed with red oaks. Burr oaks have a rounded lobed leaf, while the reds have distinctly pointed lobes. These oaks are clustered among grassy patches along both sides of the trail. Some red pines are also part of this tree mix common to Minnesota's transitional forest boundaries between the prairies and the northern boreal forest. Interpretive signs along the trail describe the area's flora and fauna.

The trail winds to the left at about mile 0.5 and goes through a cluster of red pines (with red, scaly bark) as it continues around the back of the Bunker Beach area. You can't help but hear the frolicking, playful laughter of the swimmers and waders at this incredible water park. On a hot day, it could be just the detour you will want to make.

Just past the water park, you'll come to an intersection. Stay to the left and continue your hike along the outside loop. This area has more openings mixed with more red and white pines (red pines are on the left/west side; white pines are on the right/east).

Here the trail curves to the north and winds down and through a series of rolling hills. The trail dips and curves, rises and falls gently along this course until you come to another intersection to the right. Again, keep left and continue on through a grove of pine trees. Soon you will come to a road on the right that goes to the park's Veterans' Memorial section. You could cut your hike short, walk through the memorial, and link up with the rustic campground at the other end, only 0.5 mile away.

Or, rather, continue on until you come to a T intersection in the trail. At this point, turn right (east) and follow a route that runs through part of the Veterans' Memorial area, cuts across the northern third of the park, and eventually connects with a trail that will take you to Bunker Lake just to the north of this trail section.

This is the higher elevation in the park. In fact, the trail runs along a modest ridge top and continues to climb gently through the many oaks in the area. Hints of prairie savanna and more oaks greet you as you continue through this north-central section of the park.

You will also find some marshy areas in this otherwise sandy oak forest. The marshes are on the left side along with a few paper birch trees (which are more accustomed to moist soils).

The trail intersects at a T again. This offers you an opportunity to turn left (north) and head to the activities center near Bunker Lake or continue right (south) back down toward the campgrounds and the east side of the developed area of the park. Now the trail parallels the road leading to the horse stable area. You will soon come to a trail intersection that extends the trail to the stables.

Once you pass this intersection, you are heading for the RV campgrounds and what appears to be the highest elevation in the park. The trail then begins a gentle descent as it winds back down through the oaks and continues for about 0.5 mile before coming to yet another T intersection. The left trail goes for about 1 mile and leads out to the southeast corner of the park boundary. The other trail, to the right, heads back toward the main park entrance road and then arrives at another T. This trail parallels the main entrance: to the left, it takes you past the Visitor Contact Station and the entrance to the golf course and out of the park; the right trail brings you back to the parking lot where you began your hike.

There is a shorter network of hiking trails to consider as well. One encircles the campgrounds and enables you to connect with walkways that adjoin the main bike/hike path in the northern section of the park. Another network of parallel looped trails is accessible from either the east end of the parking lot where you started or from many points along the bike path in the southeast section of the park.

NEARBY ACTIVITIES

This park offers quite a few activities for the entire family. Besides hiking and the incredible water park, one of the best campgrounds in the state is right here. For more information, check out *Best Tent Camping Minnesota*. Also, you can access the archery range, whose entrance is off Hanson Boulevard on the western boundary of the park.

Other hiking opportunities await you at Elm Creek Park Reserve, Coon Rapids Dam, Carlos Avery Trail, and a few other trails within a half hour's drive of Bunker Hills. (See individual listings for details.)

CARLOS AVERY TRAIL 10

IN BRIEF

With more than 50 miles of roads and half as many miles of trails, this hike is the only one that will take you around the edge of the restricted sanctuary portion of the Wildlife Management Area. You'll find fantastic viewing of wildlife and birds throughout 6,000 acres of wetlands that are contained by more than 26 miles of dikes.

DESCRIPTION

The 23,000 acres of the Carlos Avery State Wildlife Management Area offer some of the best wetlands viewing of birds and other wildlife close to the Twin Cities. More than 275 species of migratory and resident birds inhabit or visit the area. The land area is made up of about two-thirds marsh and wetland and one-third hardwood trees, oak savannas, and grasslands. There are two major units in the Wildlife Management Area; this hike is in the southern unit and uses the roadway around the protected and restricted area of the actual wildlife sanctuary. The northern unit, Sunrise, has a few trails as well, most of which are spurs off the roadways that run through that unit.

The critical features of this Wildlife Management Area are the regulated pools and water canals that are adjusted as needed to

KEY AT-A-GLANCE INFORMATION

LENGTH: 8.7 miles

CONFIGURATION: Loop

DIFFICULTY: Easy

SCENERY: Classic marshlands with a scattering of trees along perimeter and on "islands" throughout the marsh

EXPOSURE: Little shade once out on the marsh

TRAFFIC: Multiuse trail: motor vehicles, bicycles, and pedestrians

TRAIL SURFACE: Packed gravel with some sandy sections

HIKING TIME: 3.5–4.5 hours

SEASON: Year-round

ACCESS: No fees for trail use or parking

MAPS: At trailhead at WMA headquarters and at entrance to Old Game Farm complex 2 miles from trailhead on CR 19 (this is a very good map, so be sure to take one along on the hike!)

FACILITIES: There are no amenities or shelters along this road, so dress and prepare adequately; be sure to take plenty of water and snacks.

SPECIAL COMMENTS: This is one of the best places close to the Twin Cities to see flora and fauna in an expansive marshland—and great for watchers of wildlife and birds!

CONTACT: (651) 296-3450

GPS TRAILHEAD COORDINATES

Latitude   N93° 6.075'
Longitude   W45° 18.042'

Directions

Go north on I-35 West or East to Forest Lake (Exit 131). From Forest Lake, go west on CR 2 (becomes CR 18) for about 4.5 miles to Zodiac Street. Turn right (north), and go 1 mile to entrance of the Wildlife Management Area Headquarters. Either park outside the entrance or take road to right and park at first pull-off on right.

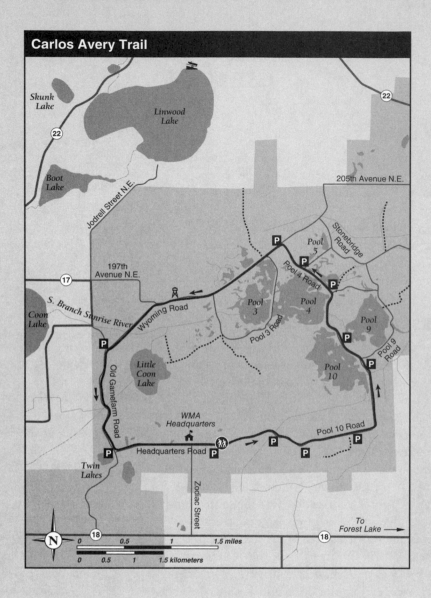

Carlos Avery Trail

provide life-giving water to flora and fauna alike. More than 23 miles of dikes contain and direct water throughout Carlos Avery. Funding for some of these dikes was provided by Ducks Unlimited and the Minnesota Waterfowl Association.

The hike through Carlos Avery's southern unit begins either at the entrance to the headquarters or 0.5 mile down the gravel road to the first parking turnout. There are a few turnouts along the roadway to pull off and park. Hikers will share the road with those touring by car, so give them plenty of room to pass. Hiking this route is the best way to see as much of the area's wildlife as possible.

The first mile or so passes through a mixed forest of spruces, maples, oaks, lindens, aspens, and ashes. Initially the trees on the left side of the roadway were part of an organized plantation planting of pines and cedars. The grassy clearings between these rows are now used to grow prairie grasses for seed, which is harvested and planted throughout the management area.

For the next mile, the road goes through a thickly forested area on the left and a wetland area on the right. In early summer, ferns abound in the shade of the moist understory, and songbirds fill the air with their calls. Expect the ground here to be especially soft and muddy during and after extensive rains. Mature red and white oaks are scattered throughout, primarily on the left side of the trail.

The road veers slightly to the north at about mile 2.25. According to an interpretive map of the area, an enormous eagle's nest is occasionally visible at the edge of the tree line. Look for a mass of branches high atop one of the tallest trees.

At about 2.5 miles, the road swings around to the north, presenting travelers with vistas of the vast wetlands that spread out across the southern unit. A drainage ditch just before Pool 10 is a structure used to control the levels of water in surrounding pools and canals. As water levels decrease in some areas, management is encouraging wild rice to grow, so it can become a food source for a variety of birds. A bit farther, there is a road to the right that can be driven or walked to access even more of the pools located farther to the northeast (several trail spurs lead out from various points along those roadways—meaning lots of additional hiking opportunities).

For this hike, continue along the main road, past Pool 10 on your left. Be on the lookout in early summer for families of geese with their growing goslings trailing behind, in addition to the beavers, muskrats, and other small wetlands furbearers often spotted in this area. The geese sometimes take a commanding stand on the roadway, but a patient, deliberate, and nonthreatening approach usually sends them quickly down the bank and into the protection of the rushes and open water.

The road passes between Pools 9 and 10 as it continues its northerly course. You may notice charring on some of the larger tree trunks, as this is a controlled-burn area. These deliberately set and directionally controlled fires help clear away dead understory and ground litter and actually help keep the uplands healthy and lush—a boost to the ecosystem. This area is reported to be a key viewing place for sandhill cranes, egrets, white pelicans, northern harriers (formerly called marsh hawks), and turtles. Check out the trees above Pool 9 for raptors keeping a keen eye out for a fresh fish dinner.

At about mile 3.5 this hike approaches Pool 4. As with other waterholes, check the shoreline for a variety of wading birds, some very well hidden by the tall, vertical rushes and reeds along the shore. Pool 5 is just across the road and a bit beyond Pool 4. It's much smaller but still provides great habitat for a variety of puddle ducks, including mallards, ringbills, teals, and perhaps even a loon. Consult the interpretive map's notes along this route, too. Trumpeter swans are known to stop at Pool 4 during their seasonal migrations in April and November.

You'll start to leave this marsh/wetlands area around mile 4.1, just after crossing over one of several water causeways you've encountered on this hike. Another prominent burn area can be seen at mile 4.3, just before a T intersection. Stay to the left and continue west now, along the perimeter loop.

A few hundred yards after this intersection, you will see a sedge meadow—a wet area "distinguished by . . . many humps," to quote the interpretive map. This area is well suited for frogs and other amphibians and, as such, is a select feeding ground for sandhill cranes.

For the next mile, continue to enjoy the surroundings, including the former wildlife management area site (check out the remains of the driveways and some planted lilacs), until you come to a fork in the road at about mile 6. Stay to the left and continue through more wetlands until, at mile 6.5, you start to rise in elevation and see a field of grass off to the right. These and other grasses are cultivated crops used to produce seed for plantings throughout the area.

About 0.5 mile past the fork in the road, cross over a small flowage, which is the south branch of the Sunrise River. Its source is Little Coon Lake a couple of hundred yards off the road on the left.

Within the next mile you'll approach another intersection. If you continue down this road, you can experience a wonderful interpretive hike featuring some history of the Carlos Avery area. This side hike will add 2.5 miles to your outing. If you take the interpretive hike, return to the intersection. The hike turns left here (east) and heads back to the start of the loop, about 1 mile away.

One could spend days walking these trails and roads, either in serious observation or casually strolling. The bird-watching is tops, and the expanses of marshland are quite beautiful—and peaceful. Take your time and enjoy this hike.

NEARBY ACTIVITIES

You are within a half hour's drive of the St. Croix River and several state parks with wonderful hiking trails, including William O'Brien State Park (see page 249) and Interstate State Park (in both Minnesota, on page 222, and Wisconsin, on page 226). Back toward Anoka County at Bunker Hills Regional Park (see page 49) are a variety of recreational amenities, such as hikes, camping, and the state's only wave pool.

CITY LAKES CHAIN,
Lakes Harriet, Calhoun, and Isles

11

IN BRIEF

This hike is a section of the Grand Rounds National Scenic Byway parkway trail system, passing around Minneapolis's two largest lakes, visiting another intimate lake for bird-watching and taking an optional side trip to a culturally diverse neighborhood.

DESCRIPTION

Like most parkway trail systems, the City Lakes Chain can be entered/exited anywhere along the pathway. You can also link this hike with several others in the book, including the Lake Nokomis, Minnehaha Falls and Creek, and Mississippi Gorge Trail hikes.

The Park and Recreation Board requests that, while going around the lakes, people walk in a clockwise direction to help maintain an efficient and safe pedestrian traffic flow. With this in mind, begin the trail at the extreme south end of the lake (where Penn Avenue meets Lake Harriet Parkway at about 48th Street), and head to the left (west/clockwise) around the lake. You'll encounter an area of small vegetation and willow clumps along the shoreline. The area on the other side of the path is mostly spacious and open. Landscaped sections and fishing docks add a rustic touch to the setting. A wooden arched footbridge just before a section called Beard's Plaisance

KEY AT-A-GLANCE INFORMATION

LENGTH: 10.8 miles, full loop

CONFIGURATION: Three stacked loops with connecting spurs

DIFFICULTY: Completely flat except for the William Berry Parkway, which is a 0.5-mile uphill climb

SCENERY: City park, with stunning skyline views of Minneapolis from the south shore of each lake

EXPOSURE: Mostly full sun; some shade along lakes and corridors

TRAFFIC: Very popular throughout summer but never crowded

TRAIL SURFACE: Paved throughout; pedestrian pathways for most of route

HIKING TIME: 2 hours for each lake

SEASON: Year-round

ACCESS: No fees

MAPS: Available from Minneapolis Park and Recreation Board (ask for the Grand Rounds parkway system); also check city maps of Minneapolis with good detail of the lakes

FACILITIES: Restrooms, drinking water, concession stands at main beach of each lake

SPECIAL COMMENTS: These trails are among the best in Minneapolis and are lit at night.

CONTACT: (612) 230-6400 or minneapolisparks.org

Directions

From 50th Street and Lyndale Avenue South in Minneapolis, head west on 50th Street to Penn Avenue. Turn north and go about two blocks to 48th Street and Lake Harriet Parkway. Parking spaces can be found in the many turnouts along the parkway. There is additional parking on most side streets.

GPS TRAILHEAD COORDINATES

Latitude   N93° 18.520'

Longitude   W44° 54.945'

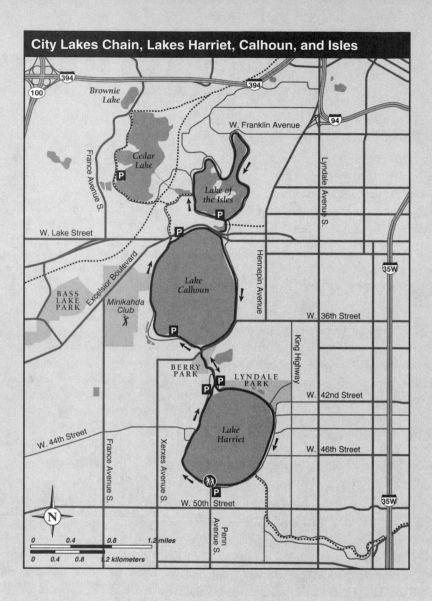

City Lakes Chain, Lakes Harriet, Calhoun, and Isles

(on a knoll overlooking the lake) completes the rustic, country atmosphere of this section of the lake.

The parkway is a narrow road along the west side of the lake bordering an embankment thick with buckthorns, cherry, and a variety of landscape shrubbery. You'll notice that all the recreational development has been concentrated in the northwest section of Lake Harriet, about 1.2 miles into the hike. The mooring area for small sailboats, the concession stand, and Lake Harriet's most famous landmark—the band shell—can be found here. Summer concerts at Lake Harriet draw audiences from the city and beyond. A great way to relax during a hike is to sit and listen to the wide assortment of musical programs available here. Some people will rent or bring canoes and listen from just offshore.

If you are continuing around the chain, you will now head to the left through the parking area, past the picnic area, and along William Berry Parkway. This pathway winds about 0.5 mile through a woodland of mature oaks and maples running parallel to the parkway toward the south end of Lake Calhoun (the equivalent of about 38th Street South and Russell Avenue).

Lake Calhoun is big and round, actually very typical of those lakes throughout Minnesota that were formed when massive blocks of ice gouged a basin out of the old seabed or earlier glacial deposits. Upon melting, they left depressions filled with water to become lakes. The path follows this lake right along the shoreline for its entire length. Stately elms and hackberries provide shade over the expansive lawns. It's mostly open air with wide, grassy play areas for much of the 3.1-mile walk around Calhoun.

Again traveling clockwise, the trail soon passes an area known as Thomas Beach. It has gone through many cultural phases but continues to be a hangout spot because of the beach and its sand volleyball courts.

At the northwest end of Calhoun looms the stately Calhoun Beach Club (the building used to be the Calhoun Beach Hotel, a neighborhood landmark for years). A parkway route alongside the hotel connects with the Cedar Lake Parkway, which bypasses the Lake of the Isles area. To make use of the full scope of the chain, however, stay to the right along the north shore. You will pass the large swimming area, beach, and parking area and continue on toward the concession stand and mooring area at the northeast corner of Calhoun. If you intend to walk to Lake of the Isles, you may want to drop down to the right and freshen up at the concession stand; there are no facilities at Lake of the Isles.

Head back north across West Lake Street and up Dean Parkway toward Lake of the Isles. The 0.6-mile-long path follows a channel between the two lakes, under one bridge, and along a built-up side of the channel. It goes under a second bridge before opening out onto Lake of the Isles Parkway at its southernmost end.

Lake of the Isles is probably the shallowest of the lakes, and at low water it can be less than appealing. However, the serpentine trail winds around two arms of the lake on the northern half, giving the hike a little more character than the two circular routes of the southern lakes.

The southwestern section of the trail is a bit hillier than the trails of the other lakes. As the trail curves around to the west side, a footbridge comes into view. The trail passes over another channel that connects Lake of the Isles to Cedar Lake. Again, this gives you an opportunity to continue on the grand tour and head west to the trail around the west end of Cedar Lake and points north. However, to fulfill the Lake Chain, you should continue over the bridge to the north.

As the trail cuts through this section, the trees come closer to the lake, providing a little shade. The trail soon swings right and down to the water's edge where a built-up bank keeps the trail from falling off into the water.

This is also the point on the lake route that brings you closest to the two islands situated in the center of the lake. Both islands are small, isolated reserves. If you are a birder, or just curious about nature, bring binoculars. Frequently, at least one of several wetland bird species is roosting along the shore or in the trees. I've seen green herons, great blue herons, and egrets along these shores.

The northeasternmost part of the Lake of the Isles is a narrow finger that sticks up into the Kenwood district. A neighborhood park with tennis courts and playgrounds is nearby. From here the trail follows the east side of the lake.

At this point you have completed nearly 5 miles of the lake loop. If you want to shorten your outing into a one-way hike, this would be a good place to park a shuttle vehicle, since there is plenty of street parking. However, persevere if you can, because the entire eastern shoreline of the lakes awaits you.

When you reach the south end of Lake of the Isles, you can double back along the channel or exit the parkway to enjoy a little neighborhood walking. Head east along Lake Street to the heart of the Lake and Hennepin districts, where you'll find gift shops, ethnic restaurants, and places to rent bicycles and in-line skates.

After you have had your fill of restaurants and shopping, return to the hike by heading west along West Lake Street to Lake Calhoun. Make your way to the concession stand, and continue along the pathway to the left that parallels the dense stand of trees and shrubs.

About 0.75 mile south of the concession-stand area, you will come to the intersection with William Berry Parkway. Take this 0.5-mile climb up to the parkway around Lake Harriet where it intersects with the lake's concession-stand area.

Walk east here (left) and past the swimming beach. This section of the beach has a windswept feel to it. As the trail turns to follow the lake to the south, you can make another side trip to the rose garden and bird sanctuary. Well-manicured beds of roses are showcased here. Naturally, from late spring through summer you'll find the roses in full bloom.

This last section of Lake Harriet offers a peaceful promenade close to the shoreline, with many spots to dip into the water to cool tired feet. About 0.7 mile past the rose garden, at about West 46th Street, there is a small swimming beach that is very popular among families with small children. It's also a major intersection with the bike trail and the pedestrian trail and serves as an entrance to the lake paths from the parkway and adjoining city streets.

Here the path is routed through a canopy of branches that form a tunnel for several hundred feet. Gnarly oaks, maples, buckthorns, and willows are the dominant species. Just beyond this cool, shaded tunnel lies another open space, along with the wooden bridge where the loop started more than 10 miles earlier.

NEARBY ACTIVITIES

The Hennepin-Lake area just east of Lake Calhoun is one of Minneapolis's most visited street corners. Specialty shops, great ethnic restaurants, and scores of handmade crafts create a vibrant atmosphere.

CLIFTON E. FRENCH REGIONAL PARK   12

IN BRIEF

What was merely an underutilized marshy area surrounded by cone-shaped mounds of glacial gravel has been developed into one of the most activity-diverse parks in the regional parks system. Hikers may want to bring a fishing pole and swimsuit along with their hiking shoes.

DESCRIPTION

Like several other urban Minneapolis parks, Clifton E. French Regional Park is completely surrounded by concrete corridors and building complexes. Still, it preserves a glimpse of what this country around the northern shores of Medicine Lake looked like long before development took a foothold.

When driving into the park, one senses the scope of Clifton E. French Regional Park. The marshes are in depressions in the kettle moraine left from the most recent glaciation. These depressions are flanked by formations called kames—conical hills with steep slopes. Geologically, this is a landscape of mixed Grantsburg and Superior Drift plain. It was formed primarily from till and outwash deposited from massive glaciers. Imagine this entire area before it was leveled by freeway

---

Directions ⟶

Drive west from Minneapolis on MN 55/Olsen Memorial Highway to Medicine Lake Drive. Go right (north) onto Northwest Boulevard (CR 61) for about 0.75 mile to Rockford Road (CR 9). Turn right (east) and travel for about 0.25 mile to the park entrance. Follow the winding, hilly roadway to the far parking lot. The trail begins at the shuttle stop near the complex that includes the boat rental area, boat launch, and swimming beach.

KEY AT-A-GLANCE INFORMATION

LENGTH: 1.75 miles

CONFIGURATION: Barbell shape

DIFFICULTY: Rolling pathway with some steep inclines; paved around marshes, beach, and boat launch

SCENERY: Pleasantly woodsy with rolling hills; southern exposure to lake and marsh country

EXPOSURE: Mostly full sun, with some shade

TRAFFIC: Promoted as a multiuse park; lots of activities all year long

TRAIL SURFACE: 1-mile loop is paved; wooded arm is packed turf

HIKING TIME: 1 hour

SEASON: Year-round; especially busy in winter due to lighted ski trails

ACCESS: No fees

MAPS: Available at park headquarters or at threeriversparks.org (look for French Regional Park)

FACILITIES: Recreation area, visitor center, drinking water, restrooms, lights, beach, and boat launch

SPECIAL COMMENTS: One of several regional corridor trails leads off the 1-mile loop and heads south along US 169 but does not yet connect to another trail.

CONTACT: (763) 694-7750

GPS TRAILHEAD COORDINATES

Latitude   N93° 25.668'
Longitude   W45° 1.086'

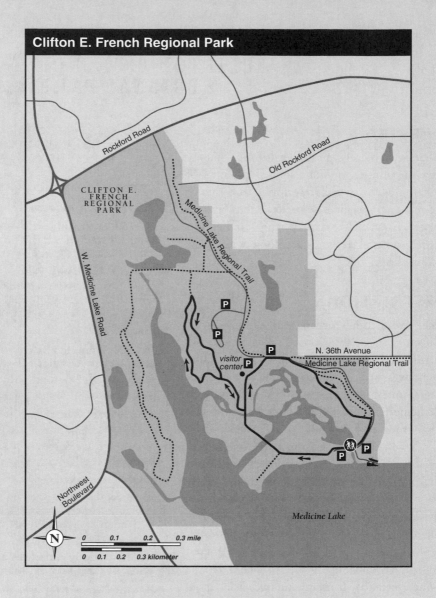

Clifton E. French Regional Park

construction and megamalls. The slopes of some of the narrow-topped ridges and hills along this hike remain quite steep.

There are actually more than 10 miles of hiking trails within the park's borders. All of these include at least a view of the park's central attraction, Medicine Lake. It has a shoreline of more than 2 miles, part of which is a 0.75-mile, 38-acre, armlike bay that stretches north beyond the main body of the lake. Flanked by marshes and steep ridges, the terrain offers hikers changes in elevation and topography completely different from the development that surrounds it.

Like most of the regional parks and some of the state and municipal ones, French has designated pet/hike trails—more than 4 miles of such pathways. These are basically aligned along the north–south ridge that flanks the western border of the park and provides a buffer between County Road 61/Northwest Boulevard and the long arm of the lake. This area includes islands of young aspens and some oaks interspersed among open meadowlands.

With that in mind, I have selected two loops that can be combined into one 1.75-mile hike that includes both a paved trail and a turf pathway.

Follow the shore of the main lake west past the swimming beach. In about 0.3 mile you will come to a road on the left that leads to the picnic area. Keep going over the bridge and over one of the many estuary channels in this area (good birding here, particularly in the extensive marshland to the east). As you continue over a second bridge, you begin to leave the marshy area and enter the steep-ridges topography between the arm of the lake and the visitor center.

After crossing this second bridge, take the turf hiking trail that cuts off to the left. This is the beginning of a 0.75-mile loop through some of the more unique terrain in the park. About 600 feet past the trail junction, you will come to a fork in the path—the high road and low road along the lake's outstretched arm. Take the left fork, which follows the low road. At the northern end of the loop, you'll see a path on the left that provides access to more trails on the northwestern side of Medicine Lake.

Continue on the upper trail and return through the same wooded area of gnarly oaks and maples. This loop section is actually a few hundred feet shorter, so you'll soon arrive at the southern intersection. Retrace your steps to the paved loop trail you left earlier, and turn left.

This paved promenade continues its 1-mile loop around the marsh area and parallels the roadway as it becomes more sidewalk than hiking trail. After meeting the roadway, the trail sticks close beside it for another 800 feet before breaking away at an optional fork in the trail that enables hikers to cut back into the marshy area one last time before coming to the boat launch complex.

NEARBY ACTIVITIES

Medicine Lake sees its share of fishing pressure—presumably for good reason. Also, the City of Plymouth's bike/hike trail connects with the park road at the park's entrance and continues west on Rockford Road/CR 90 and then south along Northwest Boulevard/CR 61 for added trekking.

Clifton E. French Regional Park has been developed as one of four official winter recreation parks in the Three Rivers Park District network. The Three Rivers Park District headquarters is located at the north end of the park. This is also a good source of maps and information on the other parks in the system, most of which are featured in this book.

13   COON RAPIDS DAM

KEY AT-A-GLANCE INFORMATION

LENGTH: 2.2 miles, plus another 0.75 mile if you cross the dam

CONFIGURATION: An elongated loop with a side-spur trail to the dam

DIFFICULTY: Flat and easy; may be very muddy in spring, even impassable in sections during flooding

SCENERY: River lowlands and floodplain meadows; great view up- and downriver from the dam

EXPOSURE: Mostly full sun, with some shade

TRAFFIC: Promoted as a multiuse park, with lots of activities all year; the walk across the dam attracts many visitors

TRAIL SURFACE: Packed earth, muddy in places; dam is concrete walkway

HIKING TIME: 1–1.5 hours

SEASON: Year-round; very busy in winter due to lighted ski trails

ACCESS: No fees

MAPS: None on-site; visit threeriversparks.org

FACILITIES: Visitor center, picnic area, drinking water, restrooms

SPECIAL COMMENTS: Another network of trails across the river is accessible from the dam.

CONTACT: (763) 757-4700

GPS TRAILHEAD COORDINATES

Latitude   N93° 18.783'
Longitude   W45° 8.509'

IN BRIEF

There are two county parks situated at opposite ends of the Coon Rapids Dam. The west bank is in Hennepin County, while the east bank is a Ramsey County Park, part of the regional park system. Coon Rapids Dam Regional Park offers several miles of trails through lowland/floodplain flora and fauna along the Mississippi's banks. For this hike, we begin on the Hennepin County side or the west bank. The trail follows the main channel and backwaters of the Mississippi along its course.

DESCRIPTION

While the key feature that draws visitors to this park is a restored dam across the Mississippi River, it's the primitive bottomlands along the riverbank that provide the appeal for many hikers.

The trail system includes elongated loops, one on each side of the river. The west bank is less developed, with trails that follow the river and provide close views of the Coon islands in the channel.

Starting at the parking lot, take the footpath that drops to the river from behind the visitor center. This is a shortcut path that connects to the river trail at the end of the dam structure. At the intersection with the river, turn right and head downstream.

Directions

From the Twin Cities, take I-94 north past I-694 to MN 252 (MN 252 then becomes MN 610 just before it crosses the river). Turn left (west) onto West River Road and go 0.5 mile to Russell Avenue (MN 12). Turn right (north) on Russell and drive about 0.75 mile to find the park entrance on the right. Park at the northernmost parking lot or at the ranger station/visitor center.

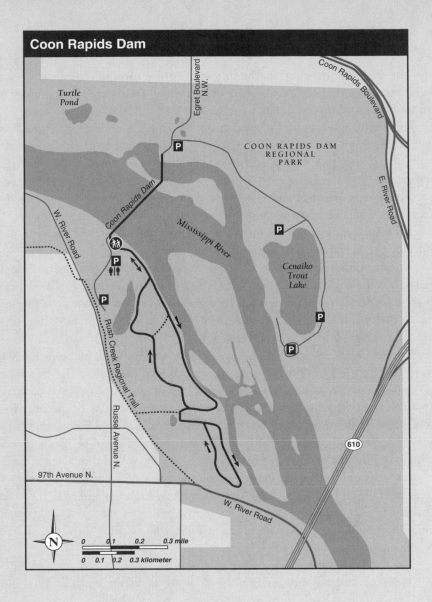

At about 0.1 mile, you'll see a trail intersection to the right. It is the other end of the big loop that continues through the wooded portion of the west side of the park. Better to stay along the river and follow this path near the water's edge. The view across the river here is unobstructed. Farther on, trees and shrubs along the embankment will make viewing the river channel harder.

After 0.125 mile, another trail leads to the right. It, too, connects back to the returning loop route. Keep on the main trail. Lowland growth consisting of dogwoods, alders, and box elders dominates the trees in this area. The path is a grassy and earthen trail about 4 feet wide. There are several thin spots in the growth along the trail's left flank to allow for side trips down to the river.

The trail continues for another 0.3 mile before turning sharply to the right (west). After another 0.125 mile, you cross a small footbridge over a creek and continue down along the stream's confluence with the Mississippi River.

The trail loops around for another 0.6 mile and meets back up at the bridge again. Hikers can retrace their route to get glimpses of the river in the opposite direction or head back through the wooded area to the visitor center, about 0.75 mile farther.

This side of the river along the bank is great for bird-watching, especially in the spring, when floodwaters push the edge of the river way up the banks. The wooded loop section intersects with the riverbank trail about 0.125 mile from the visitor center, completing a loop of about 2.2 miles.

At this point you can follow the pathway north along the river, through a small cut in the vegetation, to the western base of the dam. Here you'll see a small observation deck that enables you to get a crane's-eye view across the entire spillway of the dam. Follow the paved pathway up and around to get on top of the dam for another short hike across the river.

The restored dam uses a portion of the original dam built by Northern States Power (NSP) in 1913 to provide hydroelectric power. In 1968, it was determined that hydropower was no longer efficient, so the dam was phased out of service. Almost 30 years later, a large reconstruction project saw some of the river structures removed along with the top of the dam. This left the walkway that is used today. The dam is now controlled by inflatable gates that can be manipulated to control the amount of water flowing through, although you can't see the gates.

It's not quite 0.25 mile between the west bank and the path's terminus at Dunn Island. The Ramsey County side lies beyond Dunn Island, which connects the dam to the mainland. It provides a water channel enabling boats to bypass the dam. The park's designated amenities include a large pool above the dam for boating and fishing enthusiasts.

You can take this trip across the dam and back (adding about 0.75 mile to your trek), or you can continue on the network of hiking trails laid out along the river on its east bank. Turning south after crossing the dam, the trail departs from the visitor center on this side of the river and follows the bank throughout the entire length of the park. There are several stops along the way, including a view of Cenaiko Trout Lake and some of the development just above the lake.

The east-bank trail connects with other trails that extend beyond the park and along the river.

The northern section has more paved walkways and features stands of oaks and a 5-acre prairie restoration project.

NEARBY ACTIVITIES

The North Hennepin Corridor Trail extends west from Coon Rapids Dam to Elm Creek Park Reserve.

FORT SNELLING STATE PARK,
Snelling Lake and Pike Island Trails

14

IN BRIEF

Two trails for the price of one! Located between Minneapolis and St. Paul, this hike around Fort Snelling State Park offers a glimpse into Minnesota's history at the confluence of two of her most important rivers—the Minnesota and the Mighty Mississippi.

DESCRIPTION

The first part of this hike explores Pike Island and follows a hiker-only trail system that runs along the perimeter of the island. Whether you go clockwise or counterclockwise around the loop, you will intersect two cross trails that offer the option of shortening the hike.

It's a short jaunt from the visitor center parking area to the trailhead on Pike Island. A 0.2-mile spur from the lot cuts through a sampling of the type of growth you will experience throughout this hike. This is river bottomland, a jumble of understory composed mostly of silver maples, some ashes, and a few stately cottonwoods, veterans of many floods.

The path leads to the bridge connecting the island to the main shore. You can follow the Hiking Club Route to the right or take the other path to the left. Either way, both trails lead to the tip of the island at the confluence of the Minnesota and Mississippi rivers—the most geologically significant feature of this historic park. Deposits left during the last ice age were subsequently cut with

KEY AT-A-GLANCE INFORMATION

LENGTH: 6.2 miles; 3.3 miles for Pike Island; 2.9 miles for Snelling Lake

CONFIGURATION: 2 loops, each off a spur from the visitor center

DIFFICULTY: Easy; trail surface varies along level, river-bottom terrain

SCENERY: Mature stands of river-bottom species with continuous vistas of the river or lake

EXPOSURE: Pike Island shaded; Snelling Lake shaded to the west

TRAFFIC: Popular park; bikes are allowed at Snelling Lake

TRAIL SURFACE: Pike Island earthen and mulch; Snelling Lake mostly paved, with some gravel

HIKING TIME: Pike Island, 1.5–2 hours; Snelling Lake, 1.5 hours

SEASON: Year-round; cross-country skiing/snowshoeing on Pike Island

ACCESS: Minnesota State Park fee system: $5 daily, $25 annual permit, $12 annual permit for disabled individuals

MAPS: Available at park or www.dnr.state.mn.us/state_parks/fort_snelling

FACILITIES: Camping, visitor center, drinking water, restrooms

SPECIAL COMMENTS: Occasionally the park closes due to high water; call for information.

CONTACT: (612) 725-2724

GPS TRAILHEAD COORDINATES

Latitude   N93° 10.753'
Longitude   W44° 53.525'

Directions ⟶

From Minneapolis, take I-494 east to MN 5. From St. Paul, take I-494 west to MN 5. Go north on MN 5 to the Post Road exit; the park entrance is on the right. Head toward the visitor center parking area, where this hike begins.

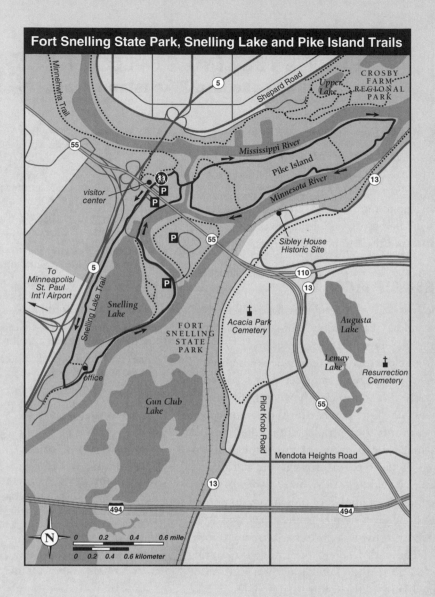

Fort Snelling State Park, Snelling Lake and Pike Island Trails

great drainages by massive water runoffs as these newly created valleys emptied out. Millennia of scouring by these rivers have created the high bluffs and expansive floodplains you see today.

The path follows the river along its banks and through a great understory of towering, broad-based cottonwoods. Some of these incredible trees are at least 5 feet in diameter at their bases. The fissures in the rough bark measure more than 4 inches deep! About halfway down the southern edge of the island, you may notice sizable gouges in the trees. These are from large slabs of river ice ripping off the bark during periods of especially high water following thaws.

Zebulon Pike, for whom the island is named, came upon this island in 1805 as part of a scouting party to establish forts along the upper Mississippi. Prior to

Pike's exploration, the area was first settled by the Dakotas who once lived throughout Minnesota. The Dakotas believed that the two rivers were the origin of life and joined to form the center of the earth.

Pike Island is typical of many islands formed by numerous braided channels throughout the course of the Mississippi River, particularly in the northern states. Cottonwoods, silver maples, elms, ashes, and willows are the dominant trees throughout this entire region. Floodplains in more-frequently flooded areas will have much less understory than those where floodwaters only occasionally reach. Expect bugs and mud in the spring and early summer.

After you complete the loop, head back across the bridge to begin the more civilized hike in the park. The trail around Snelling Lake doubles as a bike trail and is for the most part a smooth, paved surface. It's a great way to see the rest of the park and to enjoy yet another stretch of the river.

From the visitor center, follow the Von Bergen Trail south for 0.3 mile to where it connects with the bike/hike trail at the north end of Snelling Lake. Following the lake shoreline around the western edge of the triangular-shaped body of water, the trail skirts along the bottom of the bluff line that defines the boundary of the park. The trail continues around the south tip of the lake. There are two trails that lead off to the left from this main trail (either one takes you back to the main park road). Take the second trail to the left through a marshy area and across a bridge over a creek draining out of the lake, and continue back to the main park road. Go across the park road, and continue for another 0.2 mile, and you will meet up with the river trail. This will take you along yet another stretch of the Mississippi for 0.75 mile along a paved bike/hike path.

Just as you reach the eastern tip of the lake, the trail leaves Snelling Lake. There is a fork in the trail—you can continue straight ahead along the gravel trail and follow the river back to the visitor center (with a side trip to a small island connected by a bridge on the right), or you can cut to the left, remain on the paved trail, and go back across the park road to continue along the lake again, past the beach and fishing pier. Once you pass the fishing pier, it's a short backtrack to the visitor center.

The park has a sampling of wildlife, from white-tailed deer to a harmless but imposing fox snake that resembles the rattlesnake. Birders will enjoy the Snelling Lake Trail, especially the southern end, where it's marshy. Along the river, look for great blue herons, egrets, and other shoreline birds.

NEARBY ACTIVITIES

First and foremost, make a trip to historic Fort Snelling. Summer programs feature staff in period costumes with in-depth historical information on the area. The trail systems that connect with Fort Snelling include the Black Dog Trail from the south along the river and the Minnehaha Trail from the north and west. Nearby Crosby Farm Park (see page 25) adds yet another historical perspective to this heritage-rich area of Minnesota.

15 HYLAND LAKE PARK RESERVE, Richardson Interpretive Trail

KEY AT-A-GLANCE INFORMATION

LENGTH: 2.1 miles

CONFIGURATION: A series of loops, accessed by an out-and-back from the visitor center or a short spur from Bush Lake parking lot

DIFFICULTY: Easy to moderate; hilly and meandering in wooded areas

SCENERY: Winding paths through stately oaks; glimpses of ponds through the dense understory

EXPOSURE: Evenly divided between fully shaded woods and open-sky prairies

TRAFFIC: These trails are fed only by visitor center guests.

TRAIL SURFACE: Wide, mulch-covered pathways through woods and mowed lanes through meadows

HIKING TIME: 1–1.5 hours

SEASON: Year-round; access to some trails may be restricted in winter

ACCESS: No fees

MAPS: Available at visitor center or at threeriversparks.org

FACILITIES: Visitor center offers restrooms and drinking water

SPECIAL COMMENTS: This is a very expansive park with fully developed facilities, yet most of the nature-oriented trails are confined to a small area.

CONTACT: (763) 694-7687

GPS TRAILHEAD COORDINATES

Latitude   N93° 22.528'
Longitude   W44° 50.231'

IN BRIEF

Hilly islands of oaks and aspens are intermixed with some representative prairie meadows and dotted with ponds throughout a rather short network of hikes in the less-developed portion of the park.

DESCRIPTION

Though the park has more than 11 miles of trails open to hikers, I selected this hike because it is in the least-developed part of the Hyland Lake complex. The Bush Lake parking lot provides access to a number of trailheads. The paved pet/bike trails begin their 5-mile loops here and take pets, pedestrians, and pedalers in a circle around the open prairie and nestled hills in the center of the park.

However, to get a better sense of the wild side of this country, I suggest this hike, which follows some of the trails that loop out from the Richardson Nature Center and provide more samples of oak and aspen woodlands and restored prairie than other areas of the park.

Park in the Bush Lake parking lot, and go to the trailhead right across the highway. Immediately to the left, heading north along

----

Directions

From I-494 and MN 100, go south on MN 100, which becomes Normandale Boulevard. Continuing south to West 84th Avenue, turn right and cross CR 28 to where 84th becomes East Bush Lake Road. Follow the road south, past the entrance to Richardson Nature Center (on the left), and continue another 0.4 mile to the Bush Lake parking lot on the right. Access to the southern loop of the network is across the road, to the left of the trailhead for the Pet Trail.

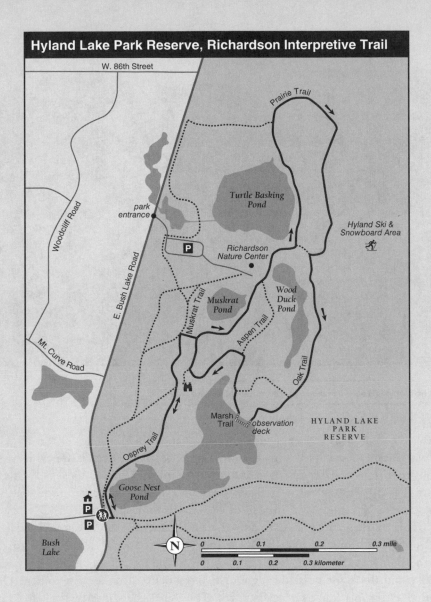

Hyland Lake Park Reserve, Richardson Interpretive Trail

W. 86th Street

Prairie Trail

Woodcliff Road

park entrance

E. Bush Lake Road

Mt. Curve Road

Turtle Basking Pond

Hyland Ski & Snowboard Area

Richardson Nature Center

Muskrat Trail

Muskrat Pond

Wood Duck Pond

Aspen Trail

Oak Trail

Marsh Trail

observation deck

HYLAND LAKE PARK RESERVE

Osprey Trail

Goose Nest Pond

Bush Lake

N

0   0.1   0.2   0.3 mile

0   0.1   0.2   0.3 kilometer

the western perimeter of the park, is the Osprey Trail. It runs parallel to a grassy path heading up into the wooded area at the top of the hill. The grass path is a wide swath through a meadow along the western end of Goose Nest Pond. Take this unpaved trail to the right up into the woods. Expect to see Canada geese from the trail leading into the wooded area ahead.

This pond is one of a half dozen scattered—mostly concentrated in this area—throughout this 80-plus-acre park. Coupled with more than 150 acres of wetlands (mostly to the west around Anderson Lake), these water habitats attract a wide variety of birds and other wildlife.

The trail climbs gradually to an island of aspens growing on the hills adjacent

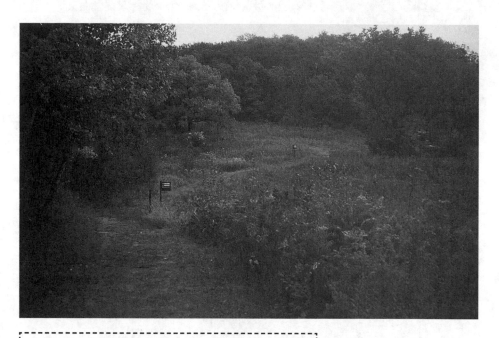

A trail winds through a meadow of wildflowers at Hyland Lake.

to this meadow. This is part of the Grantsburg and Superior lobes of the Wisconsin glaciation that occurred more than 100 centuries ago. The hills are evidence of deposits that were later sculpted and scoured into lakes and hills and valleys. More than 30% of the entire Hyland/Anderson/Bush lakes area has a soil makeup that causes it to retain water instead of allowing it to drain away.

This trail will come close to a loop called the Aspen Trail. You will come to the intersection on the right where a short spur connects to the right to the southern end of the Aspen Trail. Take this T to the left, and continue on past a small pond (look for birds throughout this segment). You are now on the Oak Trail. Stay on this trail as it heads north. There are a few intersections to loops to the left, but keep on the Oak Trail as it heads up toward the Richardson Nature Center. In this section you will enjoy a canopied walk through mature burr, white, and red oaks typical of the upland oak woodland transition zones so common to this part of Minnesota.

I hiked this trail in the fall, just as leaves of understory vegetation were starting to fall. In denser stands of trees, the loss of leaves opens up vistas not readily seen during the summer. It also makes bird-watching easier, as winged critters flit from branch to branch just ahead of intruding hikers. Nuthatches, chickadees, and flickers were ever-present in this section.

The trail continues in a winding northerly direction past a handful of smaller ponds. These are populated in the fall with several varieties of ducks, many of which are preparing for the long-haul migrations south. One small pond had quite a number of beautiful, multicolored wood ducks, the ever-present mallard, and several Canada geese that pass through the Twin Cities every season.

From the classic oak woodlands, the trail continues northerly to the open prairies between the Richardson Nature Center and the steep slopes of Mt. Gilboa, a 1,020-foot "mountain" rising out of the woodlands. This is where the Hyland Ski Area development is located. Hyland has about 46 acres of restored native prairie. Some of the prairie has been reclaimed from the agricultural fields that were created long before this area was parkland.

Just as the Oak Trail swings to the east, there is an intersection with the northernmost loop, the Prairie Trail. It loops around the east side of Turtle Basking Pond and into the northernmost section of Hyland Park. Expect a profusion of wildflowers during late spring and early summer on the trail loop that cuts through this meadow for about 0.7 mile. There are also some small islands of sumacs in this area, particularly along the southern portions of the meadow loop, that are striking in full fall coloration.

As you go clockwise around this loop, it's a typical marsh-fringed pond replete with tall dead tree snags, rushes, and duckweed. Chances are good that you will see one of the indigenous turtles basking on a log that juts out onto the pond's surface. The park lists prairie skinks, Cooper's hawks, pileated woodpeckers, bluebirds, and tiger salamanders as some of the main fauna observed here. Walking silently along the many ponds is certainly a good way to see many of these and other critters.

If you were to start your hike at the nature center, you would be entering the loops at a point just south of this pond.

As you come around through the bottom of the Prairie Trail loop, you'll reach an intersection that forks. The right fork leads back toward the nature center. Stay to the left on the Oak Trail. Enjoy more natural pleasures by continuing back down the outermost eastern loops. You will come back into the oak woodlands, along more rolling hills and wide, shaded corridors. You'll pass yet another pond, a long and narrow body of water called Wood Duck Pond. If you continue along the east side of Wood Duck Pond, you will return to the open meadow. You are now at the southeast end of the loop and even closer to Goose Nest Pond. An observation platform allows you to step right to the edge of the pond and observe the activity going on.

The trail then follows the upper edge of the basin, along the meadow and back to the Oak Trail. Take a left at the T intersection and head left as it arches back north. The next intersection is a spur out to an observation point. After the spur, the trail continues past a short spur back to the Aspen Trail (the same spur you took to get into the loops off of the Osprey Trail earlier). Take this spur back to the T, and turn left back down the Osprey Trail, and back to the start.

NEARBY ACTIVITIES

Bring your mountain bike. More than 5.6 miles of bike trails have been developed in the southern half of Hyland Lake Park Reserve.

16 LAKE NOKOMIS

KEY AT-A-GLANCE INFORMATION

LENGTH: 2.75 miles

CONFIGURATION: An oblong circle that closely follows the shoreline of the lake

DIFFICULTY: Very easy; wheelchair accessible, although pavement is uneven in places

SCENERY: Groomed lawns with open, tree-lined views of the lake

EXPOSURE: Mostly full sun, some shade

TRAFFIC: Very popular among south Minneapolitans, but there's plenty of room for all.

TRAIL SURFACE: Concrete sidewalk or blacktop in some areas; older sections can be uneven

HIKING TIME: 1–1.5 hours

SEASON: Year-round

ACCESS: No fees

MAPS: None with specific detail; all city maps will show location.

FACILITIES: Concession stand, bathhouse, restrooms, drinking water, and picnic tables at main beach; outhouses at secondary beach; plenty of parking around lake

SPECIAL COMMENTS: This is the kind of lake walk you can do over and over.

CONTACT: (612) 370-4923 or minneapolisparks.org

GPS TRAILHEAD COORDINATES

Latitude   N93° 14.594'

Longitude   W44° 54.694'

IN BRIEF

The most prominent and popular lake in south Minneapolis, Nokomis is situated right on the Grand Rounds Trail on the leg of Minnehaha Creek just west of the falls. This lake is typical of the lakes throughout Minneapolis and St. Paul in that it is a popular course for hikers of all ages and abilities. Besides its paved walkways and spacious grassy areas, Nokomis offers hikers a tree-lined promenade along most of its shoreline. Several areas are reverting back to a more natural state, providing a hint of what wilder lakes are like outside the limits of the city.

DESCRIPTION

Of all the lakes in the Grand Rounds loop, my favorite is Lake Nokomis. It's the lake I grew up around, and the one in which I paddled my canoes and kayaks and fished with my great-grandfather from England. We always told people we "lived near Lake Nokomis." I've walked around this lake during a winter storm at -30° and in sweltering 100° summer heat.

As with all the city lakes, you can start and end your hike anywhere along the pathway. I like to start along the boulevard—at one of the many turnout parking areas provided. For this hike, however, start at the

Directions

Take Cedar Avenue south to Minnehaha Parkway. Turn east (left) and continue to the Lake Nokomis Parkway entrance (signed). Turn right and go about 200 yards to the parking lot. You can also turn left at the stoplight just before Cedar Avenue Bridge. Turn left and follow the parkway about 0.25 mile to the concession area and swimming beach.

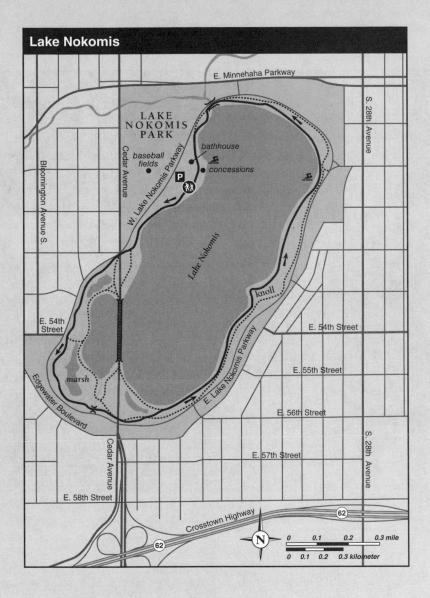

LAKE
NOKOMIS
PARK

baseball
fields

bathhouse

concessions

P

Cedar Avenue

W. Lake Nokomis Parkway

E. Minnehaha Parkway

S. 28th Avenue

Bloomington Avenue S.

Lake Nokomis

knoll

E. 54th
Street

E. 54th Street

E. 55th Street

E. Lake Nokomis Parkway

marsh

Edgewater Boulevard

E. 56th Street

E. 57th Street

Cedar Avenue

S. 28th Avenue

E. 58th Street

Crosstown Highway

62

62

N

| 0 | 0.1 | 0.2 | 0.3 mile |

| 0 | 0.1 | 0.2 | 0.3 kilometer |

concession-stand parking area. It's near the beach, and refreshments are available throughout the summer.

Head south along the wide walkway past the canoe racks and the boat access ramp. Several years ago Lake Nokomis was devastated by a windstorm that tore mature trees out of the ground by their roots. Some survived, but with good portions of their crowns lost to the wind shears, and some of the trees in this section bear those scars. The path doesn't closely follow the willows growing along the shoreline. Stop anywhere along the path to enjoy the great vistas of the lake.

At Cedar Avenue you have a choice: continue around the outside edge of the lake (the part you'll bypass if you cross over the Cedar Avenue Bridge), or take

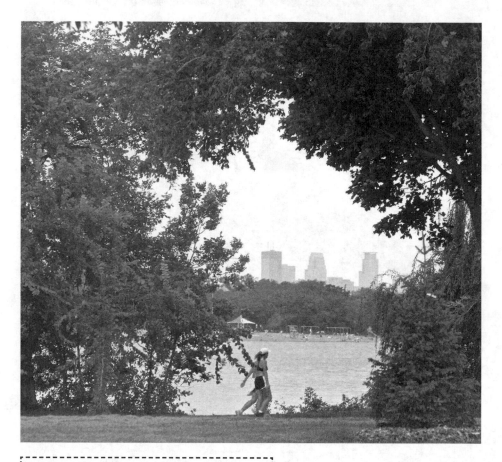

The Twin Cities' skyline seen beyond Lake Nokomis

the bridge for a loftier view of both sections of the lake. If you are into a quiet, less-traveled walk, cross Cedar and continue on the path. It leads through open, grassy areas and cuts back closer to the lake after following the edge of a wet-lands area. It then goes into a stand of cottonwoods and other lowland vegetation that lines a small feeder creek for Lake Nokomis on the extreme southwest cor-ner of the lake. This is not a maintained area—far from it at times—but it is a place to see some turtles and songbirds. It brings hikers back to Cedar Avenue beyond the southern end of the bridge to reconnect with the main lake pathway a few hundred yards after crossing the street.

If you decide to take the bridge, you have the traffic noise to contend with, but you also have an expansive view of the lake. The bridge even has a turnout platform where you can stop and enjoy the sights. Even though it's not an espe-cially big lake, Nokomis does get its share of sailboats and other watercraft—all of which add to the view of the lake from the bridge.

After the bridge, the pathway continues around the southern end of the lake. It closely traces the shoreline and meanders among the massive trunks and buttresses of giant cottonwoods. There were some majestic trees in this area before the big blowdown. Large 8-foot-diameter stump bases are all that remain of these gigantic lakeside trees. As you continue, you will start to see the beautiful skyscrapers in downtown Minneapolis poking their heads over the trees beyond the far side of the lake. There are several places along this shoreline where you can frame some lovely shots of downtown's crown.

About 0.75 mile after crossing the bridge, and halfway up the east side of the lake, there is a slight rise in the trail to a small knoll. A drinking fountain and the start of a Vita-Course (a series of fitness stations along the route with a variety of exercises you can do) make this a popular gathering spot for walkers.

Continuing north, the area around the trail opens onto a long, grassy space and open shorelines along the lake. A bit farther and you will come upon the swimming beach. It, too, is a gathering point and offers the only restrooms (portables) on this side of the lake. This beach is at the bottom of the hill of the 50th Street access to Nokomis Parkway. A couple of blocks up the hill and you'll find a little business corner with groceries and a sidewalk cafe. I think there is an ice-cream shop here, too.

The path continues around the north end of the lake. There is a section of cedar trees covering a small area where an outflow feeding Minnehaha Creek flows by just beyond the northern tip of Lake Nokomis. A small, arching footbridge crosses the outlet and continues to wind a bit through more cedars and spruce. The walkway continues through the swimming beach area and past the concession stand to repeat its course around the lake.

NEARBY ACTIVITIES

You can follow the Minnehaha Creek Parkway east to the falls, or back along the creek as it meanders through south Minneapolis. Eventually, about 3 miles to the west, you can walk around Lake Harriet, Lake Calhoun, Lake of the Isles, and Cedar Lake. The first three are described on page 57 as the City Lakes Chain.

17 MINNEHAHA FALLS AND CREEK

KEY AT-A-GLANCE INFORMATION

LENGTH: 2.8 miles (walking up the Abandon Falls Glen would add another 0.25 mile)

CONFIGURATION: An out-and-back trail, with the option of a tight loop

DIFFICULTY: Mostly level, with some berms to climb

SCENERY: Besides the falls, check out the golden walls of the ravine when sun bathes the valley rim.

EXPOSURE: Some shade up on top; fully shaded elsewhere

TRAFFIC: The waterfall and easy trail attract busloads in the summer; the trail spreads out the visitors, but the riverbank brings them back together.

TRAIL SURFACE: Roadlike surface and hard pack; the alternate path gets muddy when wet.

HIKING TIME: 1.5–2 hours

SEASON: Year-round; access to lower area restricted in winter due to ice

ACCESS: Parking lots require a small fee; free parking along Minnehaha Parkway and in recreation-center lots

MAPS: None

FACILITIES: Concessions, restroom, picnic pavilion, drinking water

SPECIAL COMMENTS: This is Minneapolis's most famous waterfall!

CONTACT: (612) 230-6400

GPS TRAILHEAD COORDINATES

Latitude   N93° 12.609'
Longitude   W44° 54.941'

IN BRIEF

This is probably one of the most famous natural landmarks in Minneapolis. From the waterfall itself and the nearby statue of Hiawatha and Minnehaha, through the lush creek valley to the banks of the grandest river of them all, this trail, as much as the numerous lakes, represents the city of Minneapolis.

DESCRIPTION

I doubt there is a natural landmark in Minneapolis more popular than Minnehaha Falls. It's always at the top of the list for first-time visitors. Prior to taking any hike along the creek below the falls, it's well worth checking out the falls from the upper walkways along the parking lot and across the bridge on the other side of the creek. You've got to see the statue of Hiawatha and Minnehaha—the love story that inspired Longfellow to write his famous poem "The Song of Hiawatha."

Once you've enjoyed the view from the upper falls area, you can descend one of the steep stairways that wind down either side of the creek into the basin created by the falls. From various vantage points down below, it's much easier to see the mechanics involved in the formation of Minnehaha Falls. The harder limestone shelf over which Minnehaha Creek flows has worn back slowly over the eons. The softer sandstone below wore much faster and the water has created a gradually expanding bowl 50 feet below the limestone shelf.

Directions

Access is available off of Minnehaha Avenue and Godfrey Road. From St. Paul, turn south immediately after crossing Ford Bridge. Watch for signs as entrances may change.

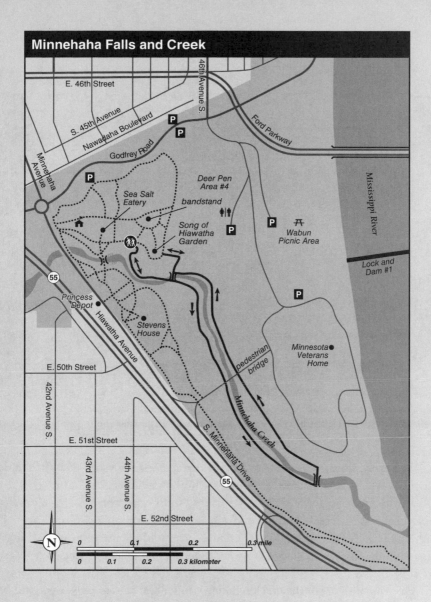

E. 46th Street

S. 45th Avenue

Nawadaha Boulevard

46th Avenue S.

Ford Parkway

Godfrey Road

Minnehaha Avenue

P

P

P

Deer Pen
Area #4

Sea Salt
Eatery

bandstand

Song of
Hiawatha
Garden

P

Wabun
Picnic Area

Mississippi River

Lock and
Dam #1

55

Princess
Depot

Hiawatha Avenue

Stevens
House

pedestrian
bridge

Minnehaha Creek

Minnesota
Veterans
Home

P

E. 50th Street

42nd Avenue S.

E. 51st Street

43rd Avenue S.

44th Avenue S.

S. Minnehaha Drive

55

E. 52nd Street

N

0   0.1   0.2   0.3 mile

0   0.1   0.2   0.3 kilometer

Just past the pool created by the falls, a stone footbridge crosses the creek and offers great views back up to the falls and down through the stone embankment and tree-lined corridor along which Minnehaha Creek continues on its last stretch before feeding into the Mississippi River about 1.5 miles south of here.

The path starts out as a wide walkway along the west bank of the creek. The sandstone cliffs on the right have seen much wear and tear over the hundreds of years people have visited this area. Old-timers may remember when a Native American in full dress would create sand paintings on one of the shelves of exposed sandstone. Today, graffiti, chiseled and gouged into the soft rock, provides a poor substitute.

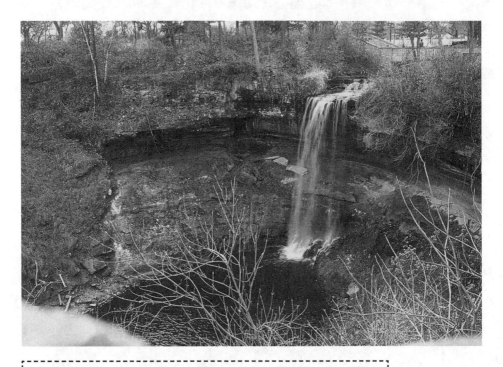

Minnehaha Falls has eroded the soft sandstone bowl beneath its limestone lip.

The creek flows at a pretty good clip throughout the year—even in the dead of winter, when the falls are frozen in a curtain of solid ice.

As the creek begins a curve to the right, another footbridge crosses it again. Looking across the creek, you'll see a long, sweeping grassy glen to the north. This is Abandon Falls Glen. It's all that remains of an old channel through which the Mississippi River flowed before erosion along the main channel caused it to abandon this course.

On your way down the creek's valley, you will be able to cross over and back two more times before reaching the river. At this point, the creek turns to the right, away from the open field at Abandon Falls Glen. You can cross over and take the wider, more traveled path along the creek or stay on this side and walk along a nonmaintained trail that gets muddy and cuts a tighter pathway through the trees. Both are very well defined, and the creek serves as a common reference point.

If you are into wildflowers, stay to the right. In the springtime, this area is thriving with the yellow blossoms of marsh marigold and several other moisture-tolerant flowers. Because of some ground springs, this trail usually always has a few muddy spots, even in the heat of midsummer.

The creek travels a fairly straight course, only casually and occasionally meandering its way downstream. The trail parallels the creek, creating a pleasant promenade between the flowing water and the steep sides of the sandstone ravine. The trail is consistently flat for its entire route to the river. The south bank does have low and high spots and requires better footwear—and more cautious footing—than the main trail.

About halfway down the trail, a few hundred yards beyond one of the stone footbridges and high overhead, are the towering and expansive steel arches of the Old Soldiers Home bridge. When you return to the top, and if you have time before you leave the park, walk out onto this structure and check out the views up and down the creek.

The trees and other plants along the creek are moderately lush, although it's obvious that the tall, lanky trees strain to get as much sunlight as they can before those rays are obscured by the high walls of the ravine. Alders, dogwoods, cottonwoods, silver maples, and a variety of vegetation thrive in this deep ravine.

Walking down this trail in the winter is a wonderland experience. The creek remains open in several spots, sending moisture into the air and creating beautiful frost patterns. As you stroll down the creek in the mugginess of summer, imagine the setting in the dead of winter and you will want to return.

The trail finally approaches the Mississippi, where the broad, sandy embankment provides a wide view of the river through tall, stately cottonwoods. To the left are Lock and Dam Number One on the Mississippi River, the Ford Bridge, and Ford Motor Company's large St. Paul plant. To the south are the undeveloped banks of the Mississippi. In the summer, powerboats cruise up and down this stretch continuously. You'll see the destination of all those people carrying picnic baskets and fishing rods whom you passed along the trail.

The last footbridge on the creek right before it empties into the big river enables hikers to backtrack along the opposite side of the creek. Both sides of the creek are distinct enough to warrant a different trail route back to the falls. Each has points along the way from which you can look up the face of the sandstone to see the unique erosion patterns in the formations. The golden sides of the sandstone cliff team up with a brilliantly hued blue summer Minnesota sky to form some incredible overhead views as well.

Minnehaha Falls is a peaceful corridor that acts as a special conduit between the activity of the city and the natural setting of the Mississippi River Valley. No matter how busy it is up top, it's always tranquil at the water's edge.

NEARBY ACTIVITIES

Besides enjoying the amenities within Minnehaha Falls Park, check out the John Stevens House, considered to be the first house in Minneapolis. There is a flower garden, as well as more overlook opportunities, farther along the upper west side. A new restaurant, specializing in a variety of seafood snacks, has recently opened in the pavilion. An assortment of funky pedal carts and carriages are also available for rent.

18 MISSISSIPPI GORGE TRAIL

KEY AT-A-GLANCE INFORMATION

LENGTH: 7 miles

CONFIGURATION: Loop

DIFFICULTY: Very easy; flat except on optional side trails

SCENERY: Full vista of the Mississippi River along entire route with numerous incredible overlooks

EXPOSURE: Western route shaded in morning, eastern route in afternoon

TRAFFIC: Road traffic; high foot and bicycle traffic on entire course

TRAIL SURFACE: All paved along main course

HIKING TIME: 2.5–4 hours

SEASON: Year-round

ACCESS: No fees

MAPS: Available through the Mississippi National River and Recreation Area, 111 East Kellogg Boulevard, St. Paul, MN 55101; possibly at the Mississippi Valley Wildlife Refuge Headquarters; or at nps.gov/miss /planyourvisit/mrtg_map5.htm

FACILITIES: A few rest areas along trail; plentiful parking at turnouts and along city streets

SPECIAL COMMENTS: This is one of the best ways to enjoy the Mississippi, the river that defines Minneapolis.

CONTACT: (651) 293-0200

GPS TRAILHEAD COORDINATES

Latitude   N93° 11.882'

Longitude   W44° 55.341'

IN BRIEF

Hike along this pleasant urban trail that follows the bluffs along part of North America's definitive river system. Pass the steepest and deepest sections of the Mississippi, and visit one of the rarest native plant communities in Minnesota.

DESCRIPTION

Almost every park in this region is tied to the Mississippi River—geologically, historically, or both. It's only fitting that one of the premier hikes in the Twin Cities takes you along this famous river corridor. The entire course of the Mighty Miss' that runs through the Twin Cities lies within the Mississippi National River and Recreation Area (MNRRA). The Mississippi Gorge section is one of my favorite sections because it's near the area where I grew up and it exemplifies all that this great river means to so many.

The MNRRA is also one of the few hiking trail networks that allow you to enter anywhere and exit at your leisure. There is ample parking all along the route, and only your time and desire to stroll will limit the amount of the 72 miles of foot trails/bikeways you can

----

Directions _____ ⟶

To reach the Ford Bridge Access, take 46th Street east over the bridge and turn left (north) onto Mississippi River Boulevard. Parking is available two blocks north of the bridge. Other major intersections with segments of the trail are at Randolph, Summit, Marshall, and East Franklin avenues in St. Paul. Main access points on the route in Minneapolis are at 44th, 36th, 35th, and Lake streets as well as Franklin Avenue. You can also enter the loop from Minnehaha Falls Park.

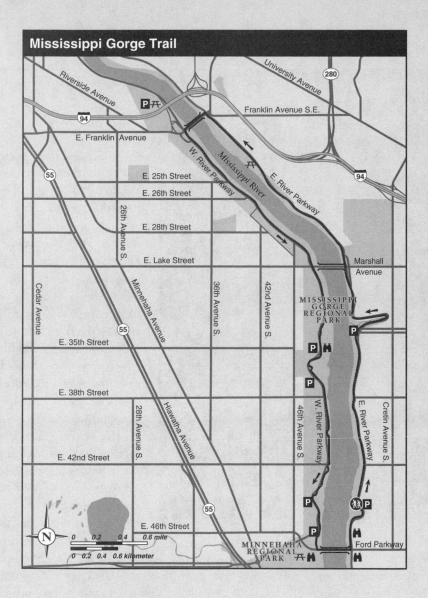

Mississippi Gorge Trail

cover. The trail is well lit, too. Old-fashioned street lamps line the promenade along the bluff, and the short stone wall on the river side of the trail adds to the quaint ambience of this stroll along the bluff. There are several places along the way where the trail opens onto a small glade, usually with yet another overlook to the river. The trail is consistent in its route—it's level and very easy.

The river presents itself beautifully all year long. Summer along any river is usually the setting for a relaxing adventure. With both sides of the Mississippi River open to hiking along the upper bank, you can hike in the shade of the western bank in the morning, and move to the shade on the eastern bank in the afternoon. If sun is what you desire, hike just the opposite.

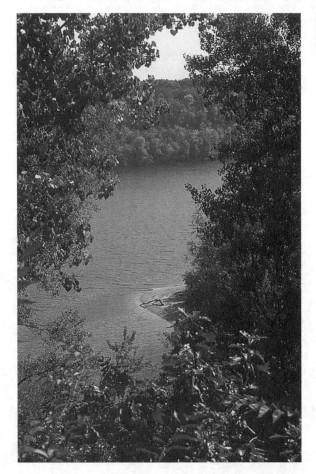

The deepest gorge on the length
of the river

Likewise, the seasons will affect the scenery along this hike. In summer, you'll find the trees in full leaf, and throughout fall the majestic oaks, basswoods, and maples display a vibrant range of colors. Winter offers the most in the way of open vistas through the trees to the river below. You pick the season, and the Mississippi is ready to furnish the perfect backdrop.

For the benefit of description, this hike starts on the St. Paul side at the intersection of Mississippi River Boulevard and Woodlawn Avenue. As you walk north along the well-defined 8-foot-wide sidewalk, you are walking the very edge of the bluff, seeing the same river that settlers have seen for thousands of years. From its source at Lake Itasca to its outflow into the Gulf of Mexico, this is the steepest section of the whole river valley. A few deep ravines have been cut perpendicular to its course, and in some spots the road and trail follow them back from the river many hundreds of yards before turning back to the main valley.

Geologically speaking, this entire area was once a great inland sea. Only the tallest of bluffs were above water when the inland seas inundated this area. The Mississippi River cut a channel through the bed of this sea to form the massive gorge it is today. Many of the other geological formations and characteristics of parks associated with the Mississippi have similar histories (Minnehaha and Hidden falls, for example).

About a quarter of the way north along the eastern bank, the river makes a dogleg turn to the east and then west. At Elsie Street, there is a small overlook that offers a great photo opportunity and a chance to capture the valley in all its early-morning to mid-afternoon sunlit glory.

About ten blocks north of Summit Avenue begins the section of the hike designated as the Mississippi Gorge Regional Park. Across the river at this point is the western section of this park. If you are interested in the history of Minnesota's prairie wilderness, plan a visit to the Minneapolis side of the river.

Just past Summit Avenue a deep ravine cuts away from the river. This is typical of the type of larger drainages that once fed the river and helped carve these deep valleys into its bank. The trail continues on past Marshall Avenue in St. Paul, offering you the option to take a shortcut and cross the Lake Street Bridge to the Minneapolis side and follow the river downstream. The trail continues north on the St. Paul side and soon passes through East River Flats Park. Farther on, past the Franklin Avenue bridge, you approach the University of Minnesota. Another section of this extensive trail, the downtown Minneapolis section, begins here.

If you choose to cross the river at the Franklin bridge, you can continue back down the Minneapolis side of the river to complete the River Gorge loop. Your other option is to turn north and head to the downtown section along the West River Parkway, an extra 1.5 miles of walking.

Heading south back down along the river, the trail seems to meander more as it follows the bluff less closely. Here, too, are more opportunities to leave the pathway shared with bikes (which bikers and hikers share for the entire length on the St. Paul side) and venture into the bluff lands away from the paved trail.

These side trails are more adventurous in spots, but they're also a lot more demanding. Most are earthen trails, which rain will make very slippery and muddy—some even impassable. One of these side trails runs nearly the full length of the Minneapolis section of this hike.

There is also the Winchell Trail, which begins right at Franklin Avenue and continues south to 44th Street. Most of the trail is paved and shared with bikers, but many other sections are unpaved. One section cuts deep down to the shores of the river. This is the most primitive section of the trail because it descends into the gorge, leaving the developed part of the trail behind for a short distance.

One of the few remaining examples of a mesic (humid) oak savanna can still be found in the Minneapolis–St. Paul metropolitan area. Half of the remaining 10 acres found in the city are located at the 36th Street segment of the trail. This is one of the rarest plant communities in Minnesota and is accessible via the Winchell Trail segment of the route.

A few blocks south, between 38th Street and 44th Street, the Winchell Trail runs parallel with the West River Parkway. There are trails off this main pedestrian-and-bicycle thoroughfare that enable hikers to drop down into the gorge section of the river.

Another ten blocks and you are back at the Ford Bridge, at a junction that will take you to Minnehaha Park. You can link up with that hike (see page 78) or continue back over the Ford Bridge to complete the loop. There's still more if you have the energy to continue south along the St. Paul side and hike the Confluence of the Rivers segment. See "Nearby Activities" below for more hiking options immediately south of the Ford Bridge.

NEARBY ACTIVITIES

Just south of the Ford Bridge is Lock and Dam Number One, which has an observation area on the Minneapolis side.

Also, farther down Mississippi River Boulevard, at Magoffin Avenue, is the entrance to Hidden Falls. This small falls is merely a trickle now, but once it probably had the roar of its brother across the river, Minnehaha Falls. Archaeologists have unearthed the remains of the giant beavers that roamed the Mississippi River area eons ago near the falls.

A trail runs south along the river from this park toward the junction of the Mississippi and Minnesota rivers. This is the Hidden Falls–Crosby Farm Trail (see page 25). It runs along the riverbank to the western boundary of Crosby Farm Park. There it joins up with the network of trails in the park and then continues along the river to connect to the downtown St. Paul and west side segments of the great river recreation area.

RICE CREEK NORTH REGIONAL TRAIL

IN BRIEF

This trail gracefully meanders through a green strip established along a small creek drainage surrounded by residential neighborhoods. The gently rolling meadows scattered along the route give the whole setting a quaint country-side feel.

DESCRIPTION

This segment of trail options belongs to a larger network of trails stretched along the narrow creek corridor that is part of the Rice Creek Chain of Lakes Park Reserve. This hike is a combination of two segments: the northern arm that winds through upland forests and meadows, and the southern section that follows the creek as it winds its way through lowland vegetation and scattered clusters of mixed lowland hardwoods.

The northern segment is a one-way, 1.5-mile paved pathway that enables you to either hike it one way (parking lots are located at both ends) or turn around and enjoy the view from the other direction back to the parking lot that serves as the midpoint trailhead for both routes.

The southern trail loops down along the creek to a gravel turnout parking lot off a service road. It then swings back north along the opposite side of the creek it follows for nearly a mile of this 1.75-mile loop.

The northern out-and-back segment heads east from the midpoint parking lot and skirts an open meadow before turning sharply

- -

Directions ———————————————→

From I-35 West, take Exit 29/CR I. Go east on CR I (Pinewood Drive) about 300 yards to the parking lot entrance on left.

ⓘ KEY AT-A-GLANCE INFORMATION

LENGTH: 5 miles

CONFIGURATION: Out-and-back northern segment; loop through southern segment

DIFFICULTY: Shallow rises and dips throughout a winding, paved trail

SCENERY: Wooded with hilly meadows interspersed along route; some sections along creek in southern segment

EXPOSURE: Full shade in wooded areas; open sunny fields

TRAFFIC: Mixed bikers/hikers and joggers

TRAIL SURFACE: 8-foot-wide paved trail throughout

HIKING TIME: 2–2.5 hours

SEASON: Year-round

ACCESS: No fee for hiking

MAPS: Online at tinyurl.com /ricecreeknorth

FACILITIES: None

SPECIAL COMMENTS: This trail winds through hills and wooded areas along an urban creek corridor. The Rice Creek North section is part of a longer trail complex.

CONTACT: (763) 757-3920; 24-hour information line: (763) 757-2820; anokacountyparks.com

GPS TRAILHEAD COORDINATES

Latitude   N93° 10.972'

Longitude   W45° 6.510'

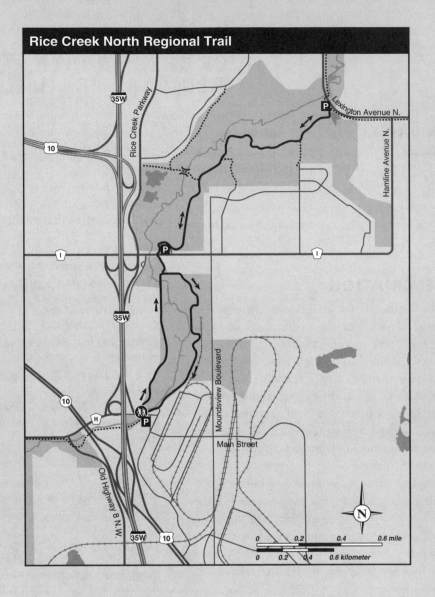

to the left at a T intersection. The trail on the right immediately joins a paved path running alongside Pinewood Drive (County Road I). This eventually meets up with access routes to Snail Lake and its trail system.

If you are like me, as soon as you reach this intersection and look to the left you will be awed by the stately corridor of pines flanking the trail like towering sentries. This arrow-straight corridor is a 200-yard stretch of tightly growing pines lining the trail, seemingly right up to the edge of the pavement. Thicker than even a plantation planting, this tightly packed, randomly planted "Avenue of Pines" draws the trail user into the heart of this northern segment.

Immediately beyond this magical corridor lies a grassy wildflower meadow on the right and a border of oaks on the left. This is typical of the northern trail

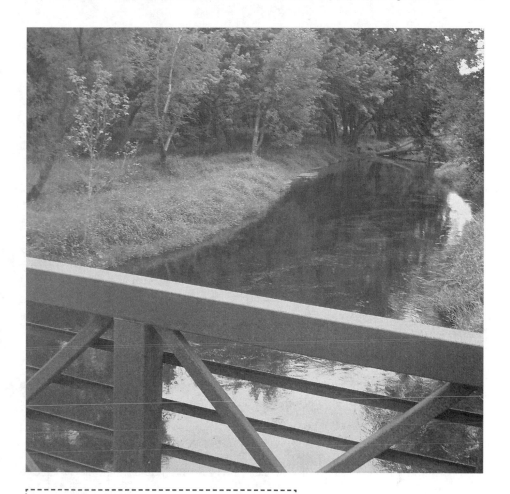

View from the footbridge on the trail spur over Rice Creek

route—small samplings of upland hardwoods and the kinds of meadows that are common where the prairie becomes oak savanna as the land makes the transition into the "big woods" forests of central-eastern Minnesota.

After several hundred yards, the trail begins to slope gently upward. You will see some of the homes bordering the park in the distance on your right. A short ways farther the trail is joined by a spur trail off to your left. This takes you into the woods for a couple of hundred yards, where you will cross a short bridge over Rice Creek. This spur continues on and heads up into the residential area west of the park strip. It's a short, pleasant side trip worth taking.

Back on the main trail you will continue northward (and easterly at times). The trail winds through more meadows and clusters of hardwoods. Although I didn't see or hear too many birds, I expect the area to have a good assortment throughout the summer, which, coupled with a summerlong bloom of wildflowers, makes this a wonderful natural trail hike for all ages. You will pass two more spurs, on your left, that head off through the meadows and serve as access trails to more residential areas beyond the eastern boundary nearby.

The trail swings north at the top of the slope you've been ascending, past the Off-Leash Dog Area on your right. It enters another dense stand of mixed hardwoods (ashes, maples, and oaks) before ending at the northern parking lot at Lexington Avenue. You can head back down to end this 3-mile segment.

Back at the midpoint parking area, the trail takes you south across Pinewood Drive and the beginning of the lower/southern segment of this two-part hike. A totally different environment than what you just hiked through, this trail parallels Rice Creek, running mostly along a ridgeline or creek embankment for most of the 2-mile looped route.

This trail may be disappointing in the scenery it offers compared to the northern section. Open field views of I-35 West in the distance and several office and manufacturing buildings visible through gaps in the foliage minimize the bucolic feel here. Still, there's lots of nature to be seen. The trail skirts the narrow, meandering creek as it weaves through dense lowland brush and a different range of trees (some ashes, silver maples, and box elders).

This section of the park strip lies just north of the Twin Cities Ammunition Plant site. A cyclone fence and gate define the southern terminus of this loop. There is a small parking area accessible via a service road that connects with Pinewood Drive back up by the midtrail parking lot.

The view into the plant past the cyclone fence barrier is of weed-invaded parking lots, gravelly fields, clusters of woods, and aging buildings in this once-productive munitions factory. Pay no attention to this, but rather focus on the trail continuing along the fence to the east (left) as you circle back along the creek and head north again.

This area should attract different songbirds than the northern half, so keep your eyes—and ears—open. This section is more shaded, too, so bear that in mind on uncomfortably hot, sunny days.

These two segments offer the casual hiker two separate biomes whose common link is the creek running through both sections. Such a diverse natural area in the heart of suburbia is truly a treasure to be enjoyed.

NEARBY ACTIVITIES

Eventually this trail will link up with other trails within the park as well as several urban trail networks. Snail Lake trailhead is a few miles to the east.

WOOD LAKE NATURE CENTER 20

IN BRIEF

This trail lies just a block from one of the busiest shopping intersections in Richfield, flanked by freeways and houses. Yet it still represents one of the best marsh areas in the Twin Cities. It offers casual walking along with lots of bird-viewing opportunities—including great close-ups of birds for aspiring photographers.

DESCRIPTION

Whoever decided to put trails through and around marshy areas within the cities, rather than drain them, should be commended! These islands of nature surrounded by ribbons of concrete offer some of the best escapes from the everyday commotion of the thriving metropolis. To understand and appreciate this concept better, spend some time at Wood Lake.

Here is an example of the marshlands so common to Minnesota, either in the form of shoreline along a secluded lake or as part of a pond in a glacially sculpted hardwood forest. Wood Lake represents an ecology common throughout this land of lakes. The trail system—laid out in a full-figured eight—takes hikers through a thoroughly representative sampling of Minnesota marshland.

The trail begins at the interpretive center and enables hikers to follow either a clockwise or a counterclockwise progression along two

KEY AT-A-GLANCE INFORMATION

LENGTH: 2.2 miles

CONFIGURATION: Figure-eight loop with outer connecting loop

DIFFICULTY: Very easy; flat and paved for the most part

SCENERY: A vast marsh with several small ponds; tree-lined to keep the eye from wandering beyond to the freeway

EXPOSURE: Full sun except in wooded sections

TRAFFIC: Popular throughout day, especially at lunch and right after work

TRAIL SURFACE: Paved or hard-packed earth; solid woodlike surface on all floating docks

HIKING TIME: 1–1.25 hours

SEASON: Year-round; best in summer

ACCESS: No fees

MAPS: Available at the visitor center or at woodlakenaturecenter.com

FACILITIES: Visitor center with restrooms, interpretive displays, small picnic area, water

SPECIAL COMMENTS: You'll find plenty of parking in the lot adjacent to the visitor center.

CONTACT: (612) 861-9365

Directions

From St. Paul/Minneapolis, drive south on I-35 West to 66th Street Exit; go east to Lyndale Avenue, and turn right (south). Drive 0.1 mile, and turn left onto Lake Shore Drive at the sign to Wood Lake Nature Center. Park in the lot on the left.

GPS TRAILHEAD COORDINATES

Latitude   N93° 17.396'

Longitude   W44° 52.862'

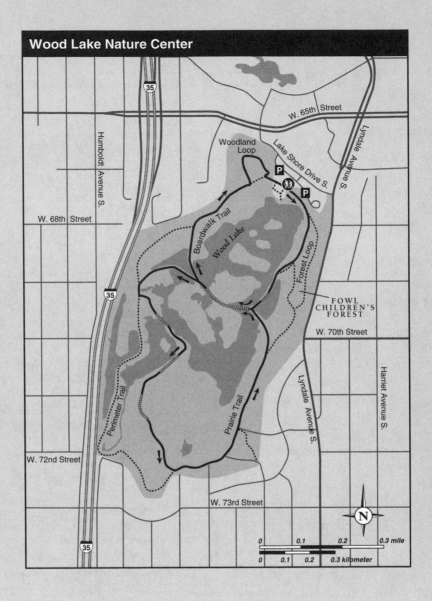

Wood Lake Nature Center

loops that begin and end at the center. A short 0.8-mile hike balloons out into the marsh and then returns, while the longer 1.8-mile trail outlines the entire park. Combining the two in a large 2.2-mile figure eight allows hikers to enjoy all the trails in the park with but a few hundred yards of double backs along the way.

Starting from the visitor center and going clockwise (south), you enter a corridor of stately cottonwoods, silver maples, and other lowland species that encircle the perimeter of Wood Park. At the first fork in the trail stay to the right, which also provides access to the observation docks near the center. (The left fork goes around the outside of the spindle-shaped Fowl Children's Forest—an interpretive area for visiting classrooms or classes put on by the center and around the outer perimeter of the park.) You'll encounter another fork 0.1 mile beyond the first one. Stay to the right and follow this trail along the edge of the cattails and reeds.

If you follow the left side, you can continue along the outer perimeter of the park. The right fork cuts away from the Children's Forest about 0.1 mile beyond the fork and connects with the eastern section of the small trail loop. This is the trail you want for the first real glimpse of the marsh.

Egrets and an occasional great blue heron are frequent visitors here, and you can usually find one or two standing as still as members of the Royal Guard. Blackbirds and swamp sparrows are among the residents in such marshy areas, and Wood Lake is no different. They are perhaps the most common of the many species in this park. I've even seen one of the tern varieties flying overhead during the summer.

As you begin your way into the center of the marsh (via the middle of the figure eight) you will be eye-to-eye with a profusion of cattails and reeds. Look carefully around the bases for bird activity, frogs, turtles, and even snakes. This area is alive with aquatic and terrestrial life. Sometimes the Canada geese, in the fall, will take over a section of the walkway; they will yield but not before a face-off. Marshes like these provide a bit of cover and rest for migrating flocks in the fall.

Resident mallards and coots are plentiful here, too. This is a great place for aspiring wildlife photographers to practice on most willing models. It's the proximity of the marshland to the viewer that is especially attractive about Wood Lake. While many of the parks and other areas provide access to and around marshes, Wood Lake enables you to actually walk through the marsh.

Continuing along the middle of the figure eight to the far side of the marsh, turn left and follow along the border of marshland and cottonwoods again. The right fork returns you to the visitor center—don't take it, though, because there's still more to see!

The interior vegetation is made up of introduced species, such as buckthorn, but the character of this border strip is that of an understory in a mixed forest stand. The tangle of understory is like that along the lowlands of the Mississippi a few miles away.

This strip of tall trees is also a good noise baffle for the ever-busy (and seemingly ever-under-construction) section of I-35 West that connects the heart of Minneapolis with its southern suburbs across the river. Like the Mississippi, this interstate is a handy connecting corridor to many more park units in the Twin Cities.

About another 0.1 mile from the middle fork, the trail forks again. The left fork, the one you want to take, swings back through the marsh and connects with the Prairie Trail about 0.3 mile beyond the fork. It guides you through a drier part of the park adjacent to the marshes at the southern end. The other fork is the Perimeter Trail. This route skirts the extreme southern end of the park and outside edge of the prairie terrain. Both trails measure about the same length.

The Prairie Trail eventually meets up again with the Perimeter Trail. Turn left and continue back along the last half of the big loop, once again encountering the big trees. Deer have been spotted here. There are numerous trails through the undergrowth, even though they border on some homes. The trail leaves the marshes and openness and flows through the dense forest of mature cottonwoods. Squirrels are common residents as are several varieties of woodpeckers, including downy and hairy woodpeckers.

About 0.4 mile farther, the trail forks again. Now you are back at the end of the Children's Forest near where you began. Take the left fork and again cross at the middle—or waist—of the figure eight. This is a short segment to rehike but worth it, since now you will approach the remaining section of the loop you have not yet hiked.

This is called the Boardwalk Trail. Turn right immediately upon reaching the other side of the marshes, and head out to the observation dock that extends into the marsh to near the edge of one of the half dozen ponds in the area. There is a trail through the woods that leads back to the main loop, or you can double back along the dock trail and hang a hard right at that point. At about 0.15 mile, you will meet up with the Woodland Loop that cuts into the deep woods for a 0.1-mile spur. The main trail continues back to the visitor center.

NEARBY ACTIVITIES

Follow 66th Street east about 1 mile to Portland Avenue. Go about one block past Portland on 66th Street (east), and turn left into the parking lot. You'll find another small park with a paved walking trail and floating walkway through a marsh area. There is great bird-watching here: egrets, grebes, coots, redwing blackbirds, wood ducks, and Canada geese.

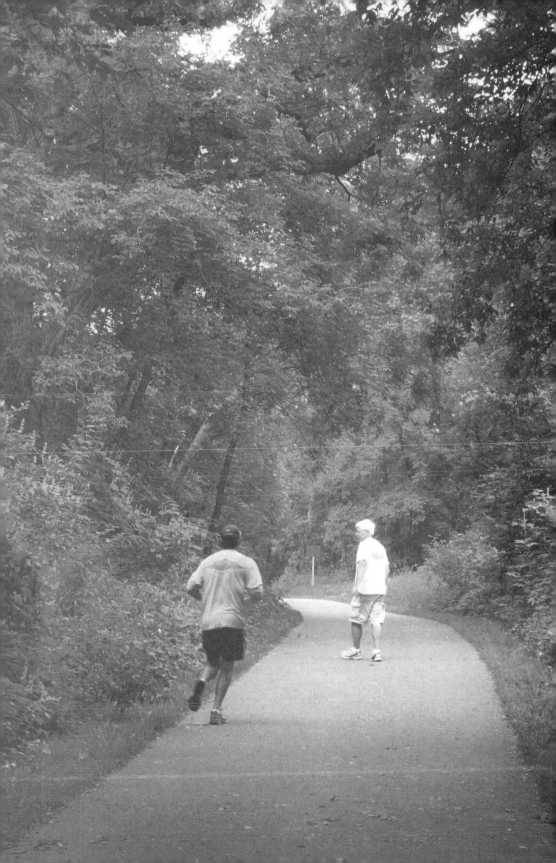

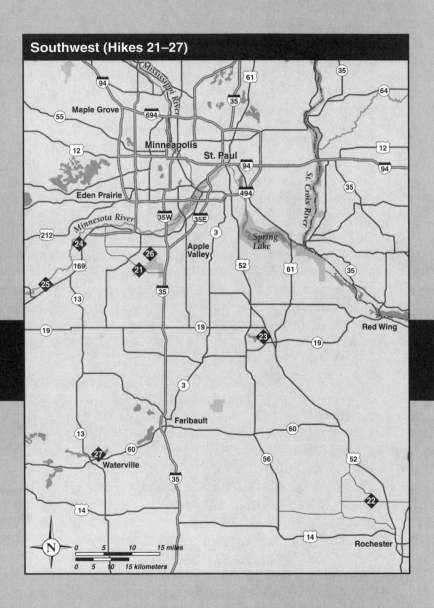

Southwest (Hikes 21–27)

SOUTHWEST

21 CLEARY LAKE REGIONAL PARK

KEY AT-A-GLANCE INFORMATION

LENGTH: 3.8 miles

CONFIGURATION: A basic loop following the lake's shoreline

DIFFICULTY: Very easy; mostly level, with gradual rises and gentle dips

SCENERY: Open country; suburban setting on periphery; views of lake

EXPOSURE: Trail is 80% open, so it's hot on intensely sunny days.

TRAFFIC: Fairly well used, but there's room for everyone at their own pace.

TRAIL SURFACE: 8-foot-wide, bituminous surface with a center line

HIKING TIME: 1.5–2 hours at a casual pace

SEASON: Year-round; separate ski trails in winter

ACCESS: No fees

MAPS: Available at park headquarters or at threeriversparks.org

FACILITIES: Drinking water, playground, boat launch, restrooms, picnic area, nearby golf course and clubhouse

SPECIAL COMMENTS: If a walk around the lake is your kind of hike, Cleary Lake is your kind of place.

CONTACT: (763) 694-7777

GPS TRAILHEAD COORDINATES

Latitude   N93° 23.221'

Longitude   W44° 41.426'

IN BRIEF

This moderately long hike around a pleasant lakeside setting is good for a relaxed gait or an aerobic workout. You won't find anything fancy here in the way of natural amenities, but the trail has that "walk in the park" feel to it.

DESCRIPTION

This is one of those casual hiking areas where you can amble along at a slow pace or speed-walk for some aerobic exercise. The 3.8-mile trail encircles the lake along a gradually undulating pathway that hikers of all levels can enjoy.

The lake covers more than 137 acres of the northern half of the park. Geographically, the park is situated in ground moraine, deposited during the last ice age—specifically the Superior and Des Moines lobes. Cleary Lake is one of the area's bigger parks—covering more than 1,100 acres—and much of it is still undeveloped.

There are about 6 miles of ski trails throughout the southern half of the park. However, for summer hiking the route around Cleary Lake is the relaxing way to go.

Starting at the parking lot, follow the wide, paved hike/bike trail north and to the right (counterclockwise) around the southeastern

Directions _____→

The trailhead is located southeast of Prior Lake. Take MN 13 to Eagle Creek Avenue (CR 21), and then head southeast to Texas Avenue (CR 27). Head south to the park entrance. For access from I-35 South at Lakeville, go west on Cleary Lake Road (CR 60 turns into CR 21) to Texas Avenue (CR 27) and south (left) to the park entrance. Turn west (right) into the park, and drive to the main parking area at end of road.

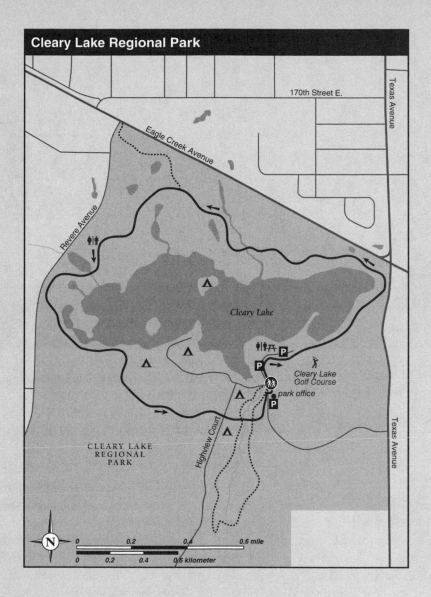

Cleary Lake Regional Park

170th Street E.

Texas Avenue

Eagle Creek Avenue

Revere Avenue

Cleary Lake

Cleary Lake Golf Course

park office

CLEARY LAKE REGIONAL PARK

Highview Court

Texas Avenue

N

| 0 | 0.2 | 0.4 | 0.6 mile |
| 0 | 0.2 | 0.4 | 0.6 kilometer |

---

portion of the lake. A small finger of land, a hooked peninsula, juts out from the shoreline right past the end of the parking area. The bays you pass feature aquatic vegetation common to lakes in this area.

The trail rises to a ridge and then levels off as it continues around the east end of the lake. Most of this area has islands of trees, albeit none at a mature height. Spruce trees beyond a shoulder fringe of grasses line the trail paralleling the golf course.

As the trail turns westward along the northern shoreline, a trail junction marks the intersection of a proposed regional trail connection. Ultimately, this park will be linked with a trail system connecting Murphy-Hanrehan Park Reserve

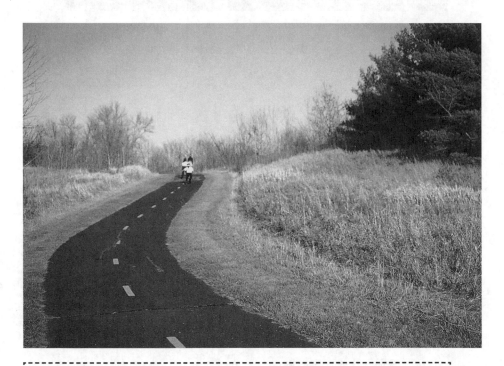

The paved trail around Cleary Lake is suitable for both relaxed strolls and fast-paced exercise.

(see page 117). The northeast corner of Cleary is only 1 mile west of the southwest corner of its regional park neighbor. This section of the trail will also be part of a longer multipark corridor to the west.

County Road 21 forms the northern boundary of the park, and the trail continues along its meandering route over gently rolling hills (with very modest changes in grade). About 0.5 mile along this segment, the trail crosses a small creek, and you'll see a marsh area on the left. Just past this creek, the trail follows the proposed boundary of one of the recreation areas that will be developed as part of the park's master plan. It will include more picnic areas, a launch facility for nonmotorized boats, and another swimming area. This section of the park also contains several smaller ponds in a wetlands section at the north end of the lake.

About 1,200 feet past the creek, there is yet another trail intersection. This is a junction with the Scott County West Regional Trail. Once completed and linked, these trails (Scott, Cleary Lake, and Murphy-Hanrehan) will stretch from just west of I-35 West south to Prior Lake.

The trail now follows the northwest shoreline as it winds southward. This part of the park is open country and a bit higher in elevation than the eastern side. The path parallels CR 87 for nearly 0.3 mile. It crosses another creek and loops around a small bay at the extreme western end of Cleary Lake. This bay features a small island. Eventually, this last section plus about a quarter of the southern perimeter of the lake will be skirted by a park road that will run alongside this hike/bike trail. For now, however, it's a peaceful route through rolling, open grassland areas.

After crossing over yet another creek—this one flowing out of the extreme southwestern point of the lake's shoreline—the trail continues for about another 1,400 feet before it turns sharply to the south and away from the lake. It cuts through stands of spruces and weaves its way toward the west-central portions of the park. Here a large woodland of oak and aspen dominates the scene. There are 4.4 miles of cross-country ski trails in the southern half of the park. One of the main access trails to this network crosses the hiking path at about 0.2 mile from the point where the trail turns away from the lake.

The trail continues for about 0.3 mile before coming to the main park road. It's another 0.25 mile back to the main parking area. The trail approaches the lake just east of the 125-foot-long swimming beach. A dip in Cleary Lake can be a cool way to end one's hike—on a hot day this black, paved pathway is going to bake!

NEARBY ACTIVITIES

Murphy-Hanrehan Park Reserve is situated just 1 mile to the east. Prior Lake, Savage, and Shakopee all offer myriad activities.

22 DOUGLAS STATE TRAIL

IN BRIEF

The Douglas to Pine Island section of the Douglas State Trail, described here, offers more vistas and variety than does the lower section between Douglas and Rochester. This hike brings you close to several farm operations as well as vast acres of crops and countryside.

DESCRIPTION

Douglas State Trail has many of the same attributes as Luce Line, an extensive 60-plus-mile trail stretching from the western suburbs of Minneapolis toward the central plains of south-central Minnesota. Like Luce Line, Douglas State Trail offers hikers a walking view of some of the richest farmland in the state.

Although the trail stretches for 12.5 miles between Pine Island and Rochester, I suggest you enjoy the 7.5-mile segment between Douglas and Pine Island. The south end of the Douglas State Trail extends to the outskirts of Rochester. Suburban development and roads in progress made it unclear as to where this trailhead is officially supposed to be.

To hike one way, you will need a shuttle vehicle at one end; for an out-and-back, you'll retrace your steps for the 7.5 miles back to your starting point. I suggest starting in Douglas (about mile 5; the 0 marker is at the Rochester trailhead) because of the ample parking, vault toilets, drinking water, and interpretive information located there, as well as the convenience

----

Directions _____

From the Twin Cities, take US 52 south toward Rochester. About 4 miles before Rochester, turn right (west) to Douglas on CR 14. Go 3 miles to the town of Douglas; trailhead parking is on the left in the center of town just before CR 3.

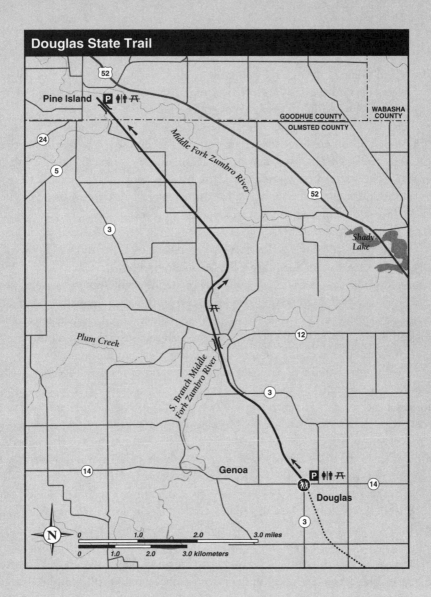

of being located about a third of the way along this 12.5-mile trail.

Hikers on the Douglas State Trail walk atop an old railroad grade—straight as an arrow for most of its length with several long and casual curves thrown in. A few old concrete obelisk-shaped mile markers from the railroad days are still erect in some spots. Those old mileage posts and the wooden trail milepost markers along the route give hikers a clear sense of the progress afoot.

This corridor is shared by those on horseback (the hiking trail and horse trail are separate and run parallel for the entire route except when they share the same lane at the bridge crossings).

Heading north from Douglas (milepost 5), the trail is a mix of open spaces and smaller trees, mostly box elders. The trail then cuts through an area of willows and sumac. At about 1.5 miles, the trail intersects with 90th Street Northwest. Views beyond the trail are often of expansive crop fields bordered by distant forests and woodlots at the edge of rolling hills.

Between mileposts 6 and 7, the trail crosses CR 3 just before crossing the south branch of the Zumbro River. This is one of several spans along the northern route that are single-lane, wooden-planked, steel-framed bridges from a bygone era. While the waters below are muddy, the bridges provide great places to rest.

The trail then cuts through a tall stand of aspens and cottonwoods, where there is less understory. An Adirondack shelter and picnic table are conveniently located alongside the trail here.

At milepost 8 (about 3 miles north of Douglas now), the rail bed is raised at an elevation of about 10 feet above the adjacent countryside. This is short-lived because the trail soon cuts a sweeping curve to the right (northeast) and stays curved for the next mile. The trail is cut into the terrain, creating embankments 10 feet above the trail surface. A dense stand of red and burr oaks and aspens towers overhead as you approach milepost 9, and the trail starts to straighten out again to the northwest. From here it's straight to Pine Island, about 2.5 miles away.

Soon after the trail straightens, you'll cross another road and see yet another place to park a vehicle on the shoulder and access the trail at this point. Another concrete railroad mile marker, number 130, appears before you come across wooden milepost marker 10. Here you'll find another bridge crossing.

Between mileposts 10 and 11, the trail almost forms a tunnel through thick stands of silver maples—furnishing lots of cooling shade. The trail intersects with yet another gravel road and then crosses another single-lane bridge. A second intersection in this stretch lies just beyond the first and features a wooden picnic table.

Within 1.5 miles of the Pine Island trail terminus, the trail cuts across the back lot of a working dairy farm. It's right off the trail so if you get any closer you'll probably be put to work!

The last leg of the trail remains characteristic of the whole route. The trees are box elder, there's a healthy understory of honeysuckle, and you'll cross still another of those wonderful narrow-lane bridges, this time at Harkcorn Creek. Just before crossing the bridge, check the sides of the trail for another railroad obelisk—marker number 127. Once you cross the bridge, it's a short shot through the woods and on into Pine Island's trailhead park. There you'll find more parking and other amenities typical of a small town's city park.

This trail can be enjoyed in either direction, and you can add 5 miles to the route (one-way) or 10 miles (out-and-back). This is truly a relaxing trail with a refreshing view of the farm country of southeastern Minnesota.

NEARBY ACTIVITIES

Zumbro River offers canoeing routes; explore Oxboro County Park a few miles east; and don't forget about Rochester. Basic amenities are available in Pine Island.

LAKE BYLLESBY REGIONAL PARK 23

IN BRIEF

Formed by a dam on the Cannon River, Lake Byllesby is surrounded by open meadows with a few low, moist areas and a small creek that becomes a wetlands just before emptying into the lake. This hike is very low-key and relaxing.

DESCRIPTION

Formed as the reservoir behind a dam, Lake Byllesby offers a city park–like atmosphere in the open prairie-and-farm region of southeastern Minnesota. The park has been developed for multiple day-use activities centered on the lake and part of its shoreline.

The hiking trail makes a serpentine loop around the undeveloped northern two-thirds of the park. Broad, mowed-grass walkways wind in and out of a random growth of eastern red cedars, most of which are 10–12 feet tall. These trees block long vistas but are spread out enough to give a sense of openness. In some spots, these trees are denser, creating a corridor reminiscent of a big outdoor maze.

Starting from the main visitor area, walk across the park entrance road to a point immediately opposite the camp store and service area. This is the main trailhead for all the loops to the north. Take this trail into the maze of cedars, and in roughly 80 yards you

KEY AT-A-GLANCE INFORMATION

LENGTH: 2.2 miles

CONFIGURATION: Loop with many lobes

DIFFICULTY: Very easy; all flat

SCENERY: Mostly open meadows with young cedar trees throughout; some plantation planting

EXPOSURE: Sunny throughout, since most trees are too short to give much shade

TRAFFIC: Casual strollers; most activity around lake

TRAIL SURFACE: Mowed-grass pathway

HIKING TIME: 1 hour

SEASON: Mostly spring–fall, although it could be hiked or snowshoed in winter

ACCESS: Fees for camping or shelter rental

MAPS: Possibly in park; also at tinyurl.com/byllesby

SPECIAL COMMENTS: There is expansive development along the lake, with modest trails through meadows and wetlands.

CONTACT: (952) 891-7000

Directions ———→

From the Twin Cities, take MN 52 south to CR 86 near Cannon Falls. Go west on CR 86, and turn immediately to the left onto Harry Avenue. Take Harry Avenue south for 1.5 miles. Follow this road right into the heart of the park. Parking lot for main complex is on the left. Trailhead is across from the camp store.

GPS TRAILHEAD COORDINATES

Latitude   N92° 56.874'

Longitude   W44° 30.891'

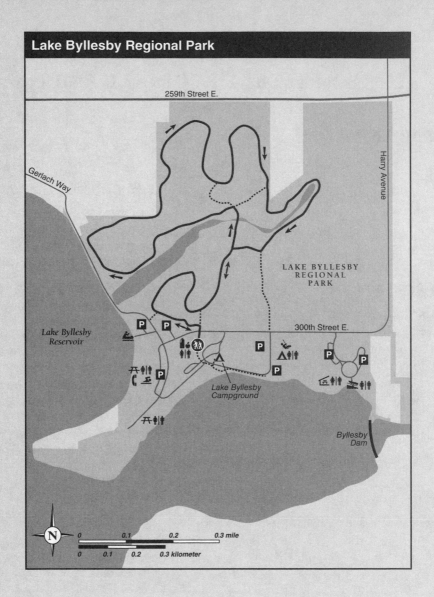

Lake Byllesby Regional Park

259th Street E.

Gerlach Way

Harry Avenue

LAKE BYLLESBY
REGIONAL
PARK

Lake Byllesby
Reservoir

300th Street E.

Lake Byllesby
Campground

Byllesby
Dam

N

0   0.1   0.2   0.3 mile

0   0.1   0.2   0.3 kilometer

will come to a T with the main loop trail. Take this to the left for a clockwise trek around the entire hiking-trail system.

At about 0.1 mile, you'll come to a side spur to the left that accesses the boat-launch parking area. This is an alternate starting point if it's too crowded at the main service area. From this intersection the trail meanders around and almost turns back on itself as it follows the long, narrow marsh area that cuts through the western two-thirds of the park. This loop is about 0.4 mile long and will come back to a spur on the right that connects with the trailhead. Stay to the left, and continue about another 0.2 mile until you intersect a trail to the right. This is where the northern loop of the trail comes back out. Ignore this trail; instead, take a left and stay straight. The creek passes under the trail, through a culvert.

Once across the creek, the trail comes to a junction. The path that continues ahead bisects the two northern loops, but you want to turn to the left. Along the way you'll enjoy some close-up views of the marsh area through the dense growth of alders, willows, and red-osier dogwoods. A thick stand of sumacs and what looks like a plantation planting of deciduous trees marks your halfway point along the marsh. As the path jogs to the left, notice the huge clumps of Amur maples. These can turn brilliant crimson in the fall. Their tiny winged seeds look like the ones you see on maple trees, only smaller.

The trail approaches a road (300th Street Southeast/Gerlach Way) that fringes the lake and then turns north. You'll parallel the road for only about 0.1 mile before turning right. As the trail continues east into the heart of the park, there are several group plantings of columnar buckthorn, locust, white pine, and others that seem to have been planted there as landscaping. Beyond the trail to the left is an agricultural field. This trail follows the outline of the park boundary and meanders along the northern block of park land.

At the bottom of the second loop, the trail intersects the trail from the bridge you crossed earlier. Stay on the main trail, and continue for another 0.3 mile to enjoy more of the open grass fields and sparsely placed cedars. As the trail heads south, it borders some private residences. At the end of the 0.3-mile section, there is another trail intersection—this one to the right—that returns to the footbridge by following the wetlands area adjacent to the creek. Stay straight and pass the intersection on the right.

From this intersection to the next junction—the last leg of the trail—you'll travel about 0.4 mile. You will encounter one last intersection, a trail that heads off to your left. If you don't want to cover ground you've already hiked, you should take this 0.2-mile trail to 300th Street Southeast/Gerlach Way), turn right, and head back to your car. Otherwise, pass it by and stay in the woods, on this trail, until you come back to the main artery you took at the beginning.

NEARBY ACTIVITIES

Nearby parks offer more trails: Miesville Ravine, Rice Lake, Singing Hills, and Nerstrand–Big Woods are relatively close.

24 LOUISVILLE SWAMP,
Mazomani Trail

KEY AT-A-GLANCE INFORMATION

LENGTH: 4.5 miles

CONFIGURATION: Balloon

DIFFICULTY: Easy to moderate; trail surface varies along gradual elevation changes

SCENERY: Prairie vistas; large, mature swamp with islands of hardwoods; historic homestead buildings

EXPOSURE: Half shaded from overstory; full sun in open prairies

TRAFFIC: Trails shared with mountain bikers; less crowded in fall; distant road noise at east end of trail network

TRAIL SURFACE: Varies from earthen to wide, mowed grass

HIKING TIME: 2.5 hours

SEASON: Year-round; wet in spring, particularly lowlands around swamp

ACCESS: No fees

MAPS: At information kiosk in parking lot at refuge headquarters in Bloomington, or at fws.gov/midwest /minnesotavalley/louisville.html

FACILITIES: Visitor center

SPECIAL COMMENTS: This textbook swamp in a prairie setting has homestead buildings and sites, coupled with historical information, which all combine to set a mood reminiscent of *Little House on the Prairie*.

CONTACT: (952) 854-5900

GPS TRAILHEAD COORDINATES

Latitude   N93° 35.863'

Longitude   W44° 44.362'

IN BRIEF

Enjoy this easygoing walk through a section of the nation's largest urban refuge, all the while passing through spectacular stands of hardwoods and swamp. The hike also winds through territory once inhabited by the Wahpeton tribe and past the remnants of two frontier farmsteads.

DESCRIPTION

Before you start this loop, read the interpretive information on the kiosk at the trailhead at the end of the parking lot. There you will find a brief history of the first inhabitants of this area, the Wahpeton, a band of Dakotas whose name means "dwellers." The trail followed by this hike bears the name of their leader, Chief Mazomani. Known as Little Rapids, their village was also the site of a trading post built by Jean-Baptiste Faribault in 1802.

The Dakotas' native lifestyle in this primitive setting forms a contrast against two homestead sites along the trail: the Ehmiller Farmstead and the Jabs Farm. The main farmhouse of each family serves as a reminder of both the progress and the hardships these

----

Directions ⟶

From Minneapolis, drive south on I-35 West to MN 13 in Burnsville; then go west to the junction with US 169. Take US 169 south (left) to the intersection with 145th Street, and turn right at the Renaissance Fair entrance. Parking for Louisville Swamp is about 100 yards beyond fair entrance (drive past Road Closed sign when fair is in progress in August and September). From St. Paul, take I-35 East to I-35 West in Burnsville; then proceed north to MN 13, then left (west) to the junction with US 169, and follow directions above.

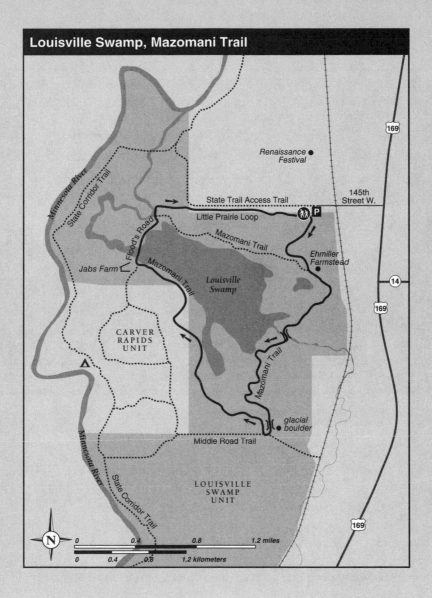

Louisville Swamp, Mazomani Trail

Renaissance Festival

State Trail Access Trail

145th Street W.

Little Prairie Loop

Mazomani Trail

Minnesota River

State Corridor Trail

Flood's Road

Jabs Farm

Mazomani Trail

Ehmiller Farmstead

Louisville Swamp

CARVER RAPIDS UNIT

Mazomani Trail

Middle Road Trail

glacial boulder

Minnesota River

State Corridor Trail

LOUISVILLE SWAMP UNIT

169

14

169

169

169

N

| 0 | 0.4 | 0.8 | 1.2 miles |

| 0 | 0.4 | 0.8 | 1.2 kilometers |

pioneers endured hundreds of years after the Wahpeton had first settled into the prairie/forested regions above the Minnesota River Valley.

Louisville Swamp is part of the Minnesota Valley National Wildlife Refuge—at more than 17,000 acres, one of the largest urban refuges in the country. The refuge winds for more than 30 miles along the shoreline of the Minnesota River before joining the Mississippi. Numerous state, county, and regional trail systems interconnect along almost the entire length of the valley. Collectively, they form one of the most extensive nature trail networks in the state.

From the parking lot, follow a short feeder trail that routes hikers to the trail-heads of both the Little Prairie Loop and the longer Mazomani (Maz) Trail. Take the

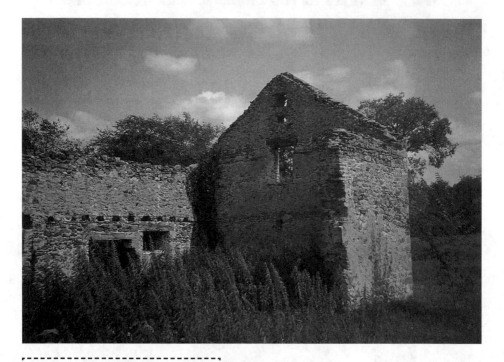

The remains of the Jabs homestead

route to the left; you can cut back along the Little Prairie Loop near the far end of the Maz Trail if you want to hike this short loop back to the parking lot.

A short distance down the trail, you come to the Ehmiller Farmstead. Its main house, a two-story stone structure, is the most complete building still standing. Exploring the immediate grounds will reveal foundations and other remnants of structures. Later, more than halfway around the loop, you'll see the Jabs Farm, a cluster of buildings offering an even more complete picture of homestead life on these prairies.

The Maz Trail gives hikers the first view of Louisville Swamp as it skirts above the edge of the prairie along a bluff. The trail then drops into the low floodplainlike area through which flows one of the drainages that feed the swamp. An environmental note: draining swamplands for fields and other alterations has depleted Minnesota's marshlands severely in the past 150 years. A project at Louisville by Ducks Unlimited is helping to control flowage here to maintain habitat for wildlife.

During the spring or after heavy rains, expect this area to be quite muddy. A high overstory of mature silver maples and cottonwoods may keep this area muddy and wet long after a downpour. Be prepared for an annoying number of bugs in the summer.

This is a multiuse park that allows small-game hunting, archery, and skiing along groomed ski trails in the winter. Be respectful and watchful of these

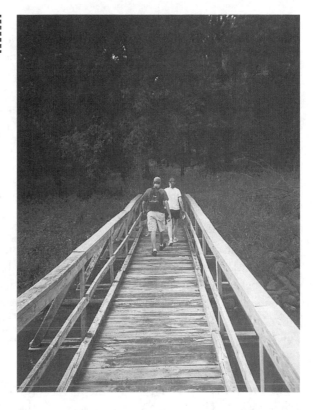

A footbridge along the Mazomani Trail through Louisville Swamp

activities while you are hiking during those times.

As you come out of the lowlands, the prairie presents itself—at least in the fall when I visited— with a profusion of late-season wildflowers and autumn colors. Especially profuse are the sumacs, thistles, and goldenrods. Islands of sumac, usually right along the trail, are common throughout the park, especially where prairie and woods transition into each other. The colors are bold and spectacular.

The trail continues southwest through hilly terrain and representative stands of burr oaks and white oaks. It then borders a marshy area that offers the first good glimpse of the lake on the right. This is also the noisiest part of the park, especially in the fall, when there are fewer leaves on the trees to buffer the sound of nearby highways.

One of the more diverse parts of the park, this trail section takes hikers through marsh areas, up along the highland meadows, and through mature stands of maples and cottonwoods along the creek.

About a quarter of the way along this trail, you come to the first of two wooden footbridges in this wetter section of the park. The first bridge affords hikers good views up- and downstream. Keep on the watch for birds, particularly during spring and fall migrations. A list of more than 250 species of birds that frequent the refuge is available where maps are obtained.

After a second footbridge, the trail turns into a broad roadway upon coming out of the lowlands. It cuts through stands of characteristic hardwoods: oaks, birches, and sugar maples. As you come to the prairie again, check out the huge boulder deposited by a glacier long ago. Nimble climbers can get a good view of the surrounding prairie from this loftiest perch in the field.

The trail follows the western edge of the swamp until it Ts with the trail junction at the Jabs Farm site. A trail to the left takes hikers onto the Carver Rapids Loop on Department of Natural Resources property. This trail loops around for 1.5 miles and features the Johnson Slough overlook. Another spur off of the Carver Rapids Loop connects with the State Corridor Trail that follows the south bank of the Minnesota River. About 3.5 miles of the trail run through the Louisville Swamp area.

The Jabs Farm site contains a half dozen structures, from a complete stone barn to the standing walls of the granary and chicken coops. The Jabs family settled this area in 1905, working 35 milk cows on the 379-acre homestead. Plan to spend a half hour or so poking around the ruins and imagining life at the turn of the 20th century.

The trail turns north at the Jabs Farm and crosses the swamp across the spillway at this point. During the rainy season or after a prolonged rainy spell, it is wise to check on the status of the spillway across Louisville Swamp. If it's impassable, you will have to either backtrack the entire trail to this point, or use the Carver Rapids trail and make a side loop hike of another 4 miles or more to get back to the Little Prairie Loop west of the parking lot.

Progressing over the spillway, open vistas in both directions present the swamp in all its glory. The gray ghosts of flooded trees and the expanses of marsh grass add character to the shoreline. Bitterns, herons, grebes, and a host of other waterfowl call Louisville Swamp home or use it for a resting site. This is a good place to stop and observe birds and other wildlife for as long as time allows.

After crossing the spillway, the trail splits. The Mazomani Trail takes a hard right and continues along the swamp, into the forest, and back down into the swamp again. This section of the Maz is also the southern portion of the Little Prairie Loop. By staying to the left after crossing the spillway, you continue up along the western end of the Little Prairie Loop that takes you back to the spur trail and the parking lot. If you miss this trail, a second trail (a grassy roadway) parallels the Little Prairie Loop back to the same trail intersection.

The middle trail (the upper loop of the Little Prairie Loop) will take you back through the upland hardwoods with a dense understory. Lucky hikers in the fall can enjoy wild plums growing along this trail. Be absolutely sure you know what they look like (little wild plums!) before you taste any. I like to bite into them and squeeze the pulp out. The skins can be mighty tart!

The upper trail of the Little Prairie Loop is about 0.75 mile long. It brings you right back to the parking lot just south of the information kiosk.

NEARBY ACTIVITIES

The entrance to Louisville Swamp is shared by the Renaissance Fair, held each August and September. Weekends will be crowded as cars line up to get into the fair's parking lot. If you've never been, it's a great experience. Also, the State Trail Corridor connects Louisville Swamp with other trailheads along the river.

MINNESOTA VALLEY STATE RECREATION AREA, Lawrence Trail

IN BRIEF

A few miles south of Louisville Swamp, the Lawrence Trail section offers more views of the lowland floodplain (high water can cause temporary closures along some routes) with trails tied into the upland hardwood forests that line this river in eastern Minnesota.

DESCRIPTION

The Minnesota River has hardly a stretch that hasn't been hiked since humans first set foot along its shores. Clearly, each of the segments designated for recreation along the corridor that comprises the Minnesota Valley State Recreation Area has ample trails and paths along which hikers can roam.

Follow the gravel road into the park entrance marked "Trail Center," and go to the right to the end of the parking lot. A path leads to the left of the Trail Center building and immediately forks. You want to take the right fork designated as the Hiking Club Trail. The left fork is a horse trail that can be quite muddy even in the middle of summer. Save it for an additional hike option on a dry afternoon.

The right fork leads through a wooded area dominated at first by elms and then by the mix of species common to this part of the state: ashes, box elders, and oaks. Within 0.2 mile, you will see Beason Lake on your left. More

KEY AT-A-GLANCE INFORMATION

LENGTH: 4.8 miles

CONFIGURATION: Balloon

DIFFICULTY: Easy; level throughout

SCENERY: Lowland; river bottoms on one side, upper hardwood forest growth on the other

EXPOSURE: Intermittent sun and shade throughout hike

TRAFFIC: Popular with equestrians (on separate trails); not well known

TRAIL SURFACE: Mowed grass, with some hard-pack earthen trails; soft and muddy in lower sections, particularly in spring or after rains

HIKING TIME: 1.5–2.5 hours

SEASON: Year-round; sections may be impassable in spring due to rain

ACCESS: Minnesota State Park fee system: $5 daily, $25 annual permit, $12 annual permit for disabled individuals

MAPS: Available at Park Ranger Office or at www.dnr.state.mn.us /state_parks/minnesota_valley

FACILITIES: Boat and canoe ramps, camping, picnic area, trail shelter

SPECIAL COMMENTS: Wear waterproof high boots if hiking any of the horse trails along the river.

CONTACT: (612) 725-2389

Directions

From Minneapolis, head south on US 169 past Shakopee to Jordan. Turn right (north) onto CR 9 for 0.1 mile to CR 57 (190th Street West). Turn left and go about 4 miles to the park's Trail Center entrance on right. Park in front of the Trail Center building.

GPS TRAILHEAD COORDINATES

Latitude   N93° 42.986'

Longitude   W44° 39.145'

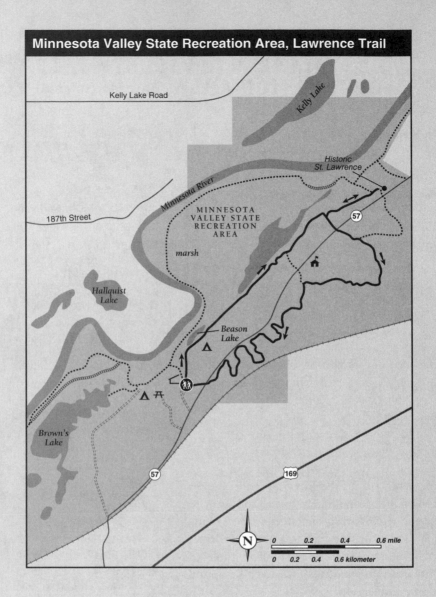

Kelly Lake Road

Kelly Lake

Historic
St. Lawrence

187th Street

Minnesota River

57

MINNESOTA
VALLEY STATE
RECREATION
AREA

marsh

*Hallquist
Lake*

*Beason
Lake*

*Brown's
Lake*

57

169

N

| 0 | 0.2 | 0.4 | 0.6 mile |

| 0 | 0.2 | 0.4 | 0.6 kilometer |

backwater slough than pond, Beason extends for 0.6 mile as it parallels this trail.

Along the way you'll pass spur trails to the left that head back toward the road and the campground to the southeast. A bench has been placed at an opening in the vegetation growing up along the lake for a restful view across the narrow waterway and to the woods on the left. This section is heavily covered in box elders, a common lowland tree. Likewise, silver maples sprout like weeds along the trail.

You'll come to a gravel road that leads to the right, but don't take it; stay on the main trail. Soon you'll come to another open view of the marsh. At this point you can see beyond the lake toward the vast expanse of marsh that spreads from the trail toward the banks of the Minnesota River just beyond the distant row of trees. The horse trail you could have taken at the fork that started this trail winds through those trees along the river.

Just past a noticeable low-drainage area, you'll see many smaller boulders embedded in the forest floor and along the trail. Off to the left sits a huge boulder about the size of a washing machine. How do you suppose it got there? Imagine a glacier carrying such rocks around like grains of sand until they settled into the ground as the glacier receded.

That would have been the scene more than 10,000 years ago as the glacial River Warren flowed through this area. It was a drainage system from the great glacial Lake Agassiz to the west. River Warren is responsible for cutting the huge valley through which the Minnesota River runs today. That valley measures more than 5 miles wide in some spots and nearly 300 feet deep.

Continuing down the trail another 0.1 mile, you will come to a meadow on the right. At the far end stands a stone house typical of those built in the 19th century. You'll have a chance to learn more about the history of the area farther up the trail, so continue on.

The trail now cuts across a willow-lined causeway over a wet drainage area. At the culvert, you are right at the water's edge of the large marsh to the left (west). This will be a good viewing area for waterfowl, particularly during the spring migration.

Immediately past the drainage area, the trail passes through a stand of box elders and ironwood trees. You then arrive at a spur on the right that leads back to the road at the ranger station. Stay to the left, and continue for another 0.3 mile until you reach the next trail intersection. You have a major trail choice to make here.

You can continue straight ahead and quickly reach an intersection with the gravel road. This cuts out 1.2 miles of hiking, but you will miss an interesting interpretive site. If you wish to visit the site, as this description recommends, turn left and walk 0.6 mile until you come to the park's official historic site, the Samuel B. Strait homestead. Built in 1857 and restored in 2000, the house is the remaining symbol of the Straits' 1,000-acre homestead settled in 1855. This and other homes formed part of a town site that anticipated prosperity from the railroad that was to pass through the area. The railroad did work its way through here, but it never developed into a stop—and the town never blossomed.

After exploring the house, you can choose to return along the spur trail or follow the trail out to the gravel park road near the southeast park boundary, turning right at the intersection with the gravel road and hiking back to the next trail intersection. There you'll turn left (away from the river) to continue the hike. Either backtracking or continuing past the house, both trails meet up at the same trail intersection with the park roadway.

You are now on a series of lobes that wind back and forth along the wooded "high country" of the park between the gravel road and the park's boundary. This first lobe is 0.9 mile and meanders through stands of gnarly burr oaks, ashes, and basswoods—typical of upland woods. The first intersection on the right will be a spur heading to the ranger station at the road. Continue straight, past the intersection, and onto the second lobe. This is a 1.4-mile section that continues to wind through upland forest. You won't notice a lot of changes in vegetation as the mowed, wide pathway gracefully winds through the trees.

There is one section about halfway along this lobe that I found particularly appealing. You'll come upon a small stand of tall and narrow aspens, their powdery white-gray bark almost glowing in the sunlight. These are thin, straight trees with heart-shaped leaves, a total contrast to the gnarly burr oaks immediately behind them. Slightly taller, but much wider, the stately oak has multilobed, dark green leaves and twisting branches that are the opposite of the modest aspen. Together these trees form an appealing contrast along the trail's edge.

The trail crosses a wet area via a wooden, planked walkway just before it turns very closely toward the road. On the left you'll pass a wet, marshy area thick with rushes (Torrey's rush), a common plant that grows very densely in this kind of marsh. Another wooden pathway, this one about 50 feet long, takes you over another excessively moist part of the trail.

At the end of the 1.4-mile lobe, a spur trail shoots off to the right. This heads back across the road to the entrance of the Quarry Campground, the main camping area for this park.

The last lobe takes the trail back across the road and diagonally through the woods as it leads back to the parking lot for the last 0.4 mile of the hike. You reenter the parking lot on the right side of the Trail Center building.

NEARBY ACTIVITIES

Just north of Jordan is the Louisville Swamp section of the Minnesota Valley State Recreation Area, which offers excellent hiking and historical landmarks (see page 108).

MURPHY-HANREHAN PARK RESERVE 26

IN BRIEF

One of the most rugged parks in the Henne-pin park system, this hike offers diverse terrain, challenging trails, and a great strenuous hike for those who want a good workout. This is a beautiful area with serious glacial moraine and one of the best stands of oaks in the Twin Cities.

DESCRIPTION

With two networks of hiking trails (this hike takes place in only the north section), Murphy-Hanrehan Park Reserve offers some of the most challenging terrain for hiking of all the parks in the region.

The northern section of the park, east of County Road 75, contains about half of the 18.2 miles of hiking trails within the park. The extreme northeast trail network in this part, numbered 4–9 on the trail map, are open to hiking August–November only. All the mountain-biking trails are now across the road (CR 75) in their own section with their own network of trails.

What makes this park topographically challenging are the steep glacial deposits—moraines—upon which this land developed.

Directions ⟶

The park lies south of Savage and west of Burnsville. Take I-35 East from St. Paul or I-35 West from Minneapolis to Burnsville. Take Exit 88B onto CR 42. Go west 2 miles to Hanrehan Lake Boulevard (CR 74). Turn left and go west 2 miles to Murphy Lake Boulevard (CR 75). The entrance is on the left. Look for the parking area and trailhead on the left, just inside the park. The turnout and gate for the alternate hike (Trail 12) are about 0.5 mile farther on left.

i KEY AT-A-GLANCE INFORMATION

LENGTH: 1.5 miles; alternate route, 4.5 miles; total trail mile options, 18.2 miles

CONFIGURATION: Balloon; alternate trail similar with options

DIFFICULTY: Moderate to moderately difficult on steeper sections

SCENERY: Very hilly, with a solid stand of oaks

EXPOSURE: Mostly shaded, with some sun near the main trailhead

TRAFFIC: Except during winter cross-country skiing and spring mountain-bike seasons, it could be very tranquil.

TRAIL SURFACE: Packed earth, though horse trails are a bit soft; biking trails are well worn; also some exposed rocks and roots.

HIKING TIME: Main trail, 45 minutes; alternate trail, 2–2.5 hours

SEASON: Early spring for least amount of alternative trail use

ACCESS: No fees

MAPS: Possibly at park and at threeriversparks.org

FACILITIES: Pit toilet, drinking water

SPECIAL COMMENTS: The best trails must be shared with other users.

CONTACT: (763) 694-7777

GPS TRAILHEAD COORDINATES

Latitude   N93° 20.869'
Longitude   W44° 43.450'

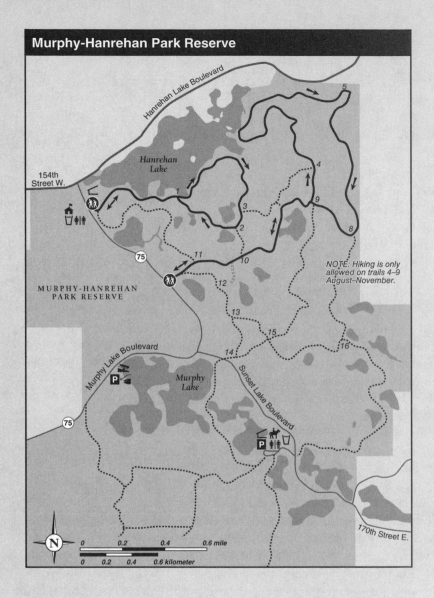

Murphy-Hanrehan Park Reserve

These moraines were formed during the fifth (and last) Wisconsin glacial period. This created a landscape pockmarked with sandy, conical-shaped hills called kames. Elevations in the park vary by more than 100 feet. In addition to these hills, myriad lakes, ponds, and marshy areas have developed in the lowlands. The basins formed by the steep-sided kames are called kettles.

From the parking area at the entrance off of Hanrehan Boulevard, hike east and then take the left fork of the trail (Trail 1) and follow along the level ground south of Hanrehan Lake for 0.3 mile. The trail then forks again—stay left and start a climb toward the top of one of scores of kames in the park. The lowlands around the lake give way to impressive stands of oaks—one of the other natural features of this park besides remnants of the past ice age.

The predominant forest is composed of oak mixed with aspen. This growth is limited to the ridges and encircles some of the marshy areas. Open prairielike meadows are more a southern park feature.

The trail simply loops back around for about 0.5 mile to intersect with Trail 3 (posted). Take a right, which will lead you back to the first fork from the parking area. You must retrace your steps for the last 0.4 mile back to the trailhead.

However, here is a great alternate route to consider: instead of taking Trail 1 from the trailhead, hang a right onto Trail 11. You can follow this trail east to the intersection with Trail 10. Trail 10 continues to the right and will connect with the 4–9 trail loop, open for hiking August–November only, farther on.

Be on the lookout for some rare glimpses of visiting songbirds and raptors. The park boasts an impressive bird list: loons, red-shouldered hawks, and two species of night herons. Other birds to look for are the rare Arcadian flycatcher, Bell's vireo (another rarely seen bird), and scarlet tanagers. Also calling the park home are owls, mink woodpeckers, foxes, coyotes, and wild turkeys.

Trail 10 winds through stately stands of oaks without a lot of understory. There are kettles in many places along the route as the trail twists around them or climbs to the top of one of the kames. At the intersection with Trail 9, take a left and start hiking on Trail 4. This route is even more strenuous than before, but the corridors are wide and easy to walk. This trail cuts a serpentine swath through oaks growing high on the series of ridges formed above the northeast end of Hanrehan Lake. The trail does several severe cuts back and forth before a long drop toward the lake. It continues around in a mile-long loop passing intersections with Trails 5, 6, 7, and 8 before connecting with Trail 9 again.

In the summer you can continue along one of the cross-country ski trails (if open). Both Trails 9 and 10 provide a longer loop that connects back to the corridor made by Trail 13, which in turn leads back to the road. Otherwise, you will need to return along Trail 9, past the intersection with Trail 4, and head back out the way you came in. I strongly advise hikers to carry a map. Without one, you can take quite a few extra steps and turns before arriving at a familiar crossing. With a map, this tangle of turning trails coupled with hills and ponds can be one of the most rewarding hiking areas for sheer challenge alone. You will find plenty of opportunities to test your leg muscles in this park.

NEARBY ACTIVITIES

The southern section of Murphy-Hanrehan Park Reserve has another network of hiking trails, including a loop around Minnregs Lake at the southeastern corner. You are also within a mile of Cleary Lake. Modern and tame compared to Murphy-Hanrehan's ruggedness, it's close enough to be a great after-hiking area in which to picnic or casually stretch out your muscles using the paved hiking pathway.

27 SAKATAH LAKE STATE PARK

KEY AT-A-GLANCE INFORMATION

LENGTH: 2.2 miles

CONFIGURATION: Two stacked loops

DIFFICULTY: Easy to moderate; portions are level and easy, while others make a moderate climb to a 100-foot change in elevation.

SCENERY: Big-woods feeling with a long view down a very narrow corridor

EXPOSURE: Mostly shade

TRAFFIC: State trail busy with bike traffic in summer and snow machines in winter

TRAIL SURFACE: State trail is wide, paved surface; within park are narrow, earthen trails.

HIKING TIME: 1–1.5 hours

SEASON: Year-round; spring for birds, fall for colors, winter for skiing

ACCESS: Minnesota State Park fee system: $5 daily, $25 annual permit, $12 annual permit for disabled persons

MAPS: Available at park headquarters or at www.dnr.state.mn.us /state_parks/sakatah_lake

FACILITIES: Interpretive center, restrooms, showers, drinking water

SPECIAL COMMENTS: Hiking and lakeside/boating activities offer much for everyone.

CONTACT: (507) 362-4438

GPS TRAILHEAD COORDINATES

Latitude   N93° 31.924'

Longitude   W44° 13.235'

IN BRIEF

The Dakota tribe of Wahpekita Native Americans called this area Sakatah, or "Singing Hills." The area represents the transition zone between the "big woods" and more open southern Minnesota prairie.

DESCRIPTION

There are two trail systems to consider at Sakatah Lake State Park: the trails within the park and the 39-mile Singing Hills State Trail corridor that's part of the state's system of converted railroad-bed trails. This particular corridor links the towns of Mankato and Faribault. Hoping to capture the flavor of each, I've incorporated a hike that forms an irregular loop encompassing both.

From the interpretive center, hook up with the campground access trail that heads down to the lake via a 0.3-mile trail. At about 0.2 mile, this trail intersects one of the park's main hiking trails, the Oak Tree Trail. This intersection comes just before the final downhill path to the Singing Hills Trail.

You can't miss the Singing Hills Trail. This old railroad bed creates a wide, canopied corridor as it parallels the shores of Sakatah Lake—a widening in the Cannon River. Take a left (west), and head down the trail.

You hit the Wahpekita Trail 0.2 mile farther, which is a 0.6-mile trail along the lakeshore to the fishing pier and lakeside picnic grounds.

Directions ⟶

From the Twin Cities, take I-35 south to Faribault (Exit 56); then go about 12 miles west of Faribault on MN 60. Turn right at the park entrance, and take the next left to park near the interpretive center.

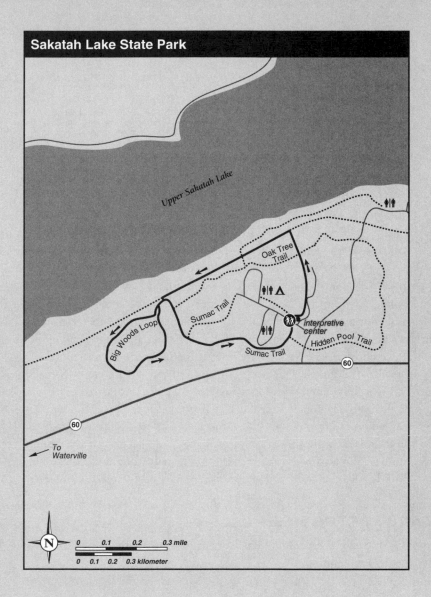

By staying on the Singing Hills Trail, hikers can enjoy a paved, 8-foot-wide pathway that is as straight as an arrow—or at least as a former train track. Abandoned in the early 1970s, this used to be the route taken by the Chicago & North Western Railway. However, to enjoy the park's trails you must leave the Singing Hills Trail at this intersection and take the trail to the left. This leads to the T intersection with the Oak Tree Trail. Take the Oak Tree Trail to the right. It parallels the railroad bed but allows you to continue hiking on trails within the park.

Continue on the Oak Tree Trail for about 0.3 mile to another T intersection, this time with the Sumac Trail. Follow the Sumac Trail to the right, and cross the bridge over the creek less than 0.1 mile farther. You will be at the beginning of the

Big Woods Loop Trail just after you cross this bridge. Take the right fork, and walk the loop counterclockwise.

The park has given this loop trail a Sioux name as well: "Tanka Canwitc." I've seen enough movies to convince me that *tanka* means "big." The Big Woods Loop is a 0.7-mile climb up and through the mature oaks and maples characteristic of the big-woods forests that once covered this portion of Minnesota. This area is what's called an ecotone—a transition zone between the Southern Oak Barrens and the Big Woods landscape regions.

Geologically speaking, this area was sculpted most recently by glacial activity about 14,000 years ago. A large glacial deposit, a moraine made up of rock and up to 400 feet deep, was laid down over the existing bedrock. As the glaciers receded, large chunks of ice were shoved into the ground. These melted, forming the basins of lakes in the area, including Sakatah and Lower Sakatah lakes.

Coming down off the loop, you will need to retrace your steps back over the bridge and continue south farther away from the lake. Ignore the first intersection, which is actually the west end of Oak Tree Trail. Instead, continue along the southerly trail for about 0.15 mile. You are now at the intersection with Sumac Trail.

Instead of taking the left trail, continue ahead to the south for about 0.5 mile. This is a hilly climb with lots of oak and maple understory. The woodland you pass through developed after the Wisconsin ice age. This is the same look the forest had when the first non–Native American settlers began arriving.

You'll approach another trail junction toward the end of the Sumac Trail. This is Lower Sumac Trail. It leads back to the main road and access to Hidden Pond Trail. Ignore this option, and continue that last bit back to your car.

NEARBY ACTIVITIES

The Sakatah Singing Hills State Trail extends west 22 miles to Mankato or 14 miles east to Faribault.

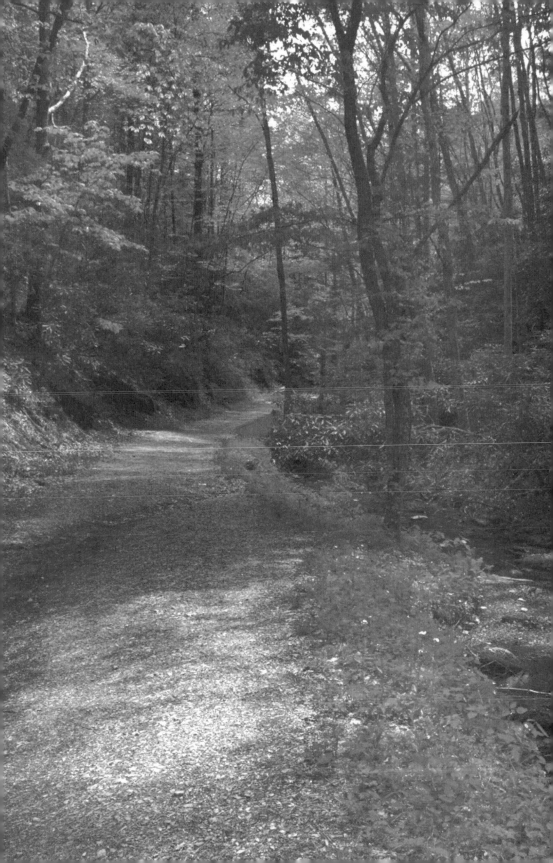

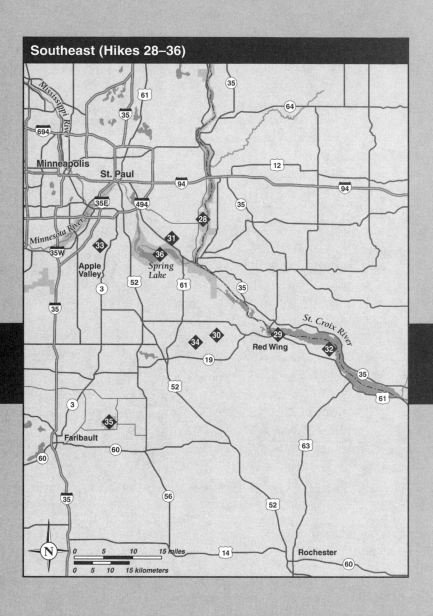

Southeast (Hikes 28–36)

SOUTHEAST

28 AFTON STATE PARK

KEY AT-A-GLANCE INFORMATION

LENGTH: 4.3 miles

CONFIGURATION: Balloon

DIFFICULTY: Moderate to strenuous due to elevation changes exceeding 300 feet in less than 0.5 mile; easy along upper meadows and lowlands

SCENERY: Mature oak forests, delicate prairies, ravines, and impressive vistas of the St. Croix River

EXPOSURE: Fully exposed meadows atop bluffs; dense canopies in ravines

TRAFFIC: Popular with hikers; beaches get crowded in summer.

TRAIL SURFACE: Paved surface, wide grassy lanes, and narrow, uneven surfaces along ravines

HIKING TIME: 2 hours

SEASON: Year-round; many trails are converted for cross-country skiing.

ACCESS: Minnesota State Park fee system: $5 daily, $25 annual permit, or $12 annual permit for disabled individuals

MAPS: Available at park or at www .dnr.state.mn.us/state_parks/afton

FACILITIES: Developed campsites, picnic areas, restrooms, beach, and interpretive center

SPECIAL COMMENTS: Great for weekend campers and hikers.

CONTACT: (651) 436-5391

GPS TRAILHEAD COORDINATES

Latitude   N92° 46.362'

Longitude   W44° 50.760'

IN BRIEF

More than 20 miles of trails crisscross oak savannas and follow ravines cut deeper than 300 feet into the bluffs of the St. Croix River. This park provides hikers with serious trails, expansive river beaches, and myriad vistas of the beautiful St. Croix River and valley.

DESCRIPTION

The main trail leaving from the parking lot at Afton State Park is like a promenade leading to the main activity areas of the park. Its wide, paved path leads hikers down an incline along a gradually winding trail past the picnic area and group sites atop a wooded ridge above the river. The ridgetop trail ends at a series of steps that drop the trail quickly to the lowlands along the river. There it continues through lowland forests of spindly maples, ironwoods, ashes, and a dense understory. The trail crosses an unnamed creek (great for wading on those hot, humid days of summer) and opens onto the main path, an old railroad grade that serves as the main trail along the river, before bringing trekkers onto the lower picnic and beach area along the St. Croix River.

At this intersection, hiking trails weave out to the north and west to join up with a web of trails in the northern region of Afton State Park.

Directions ⟶

From downtown St. Paul, head east on I-94 for 9 miles to CR 15/MN 95 (Exit 253). Go south 7 miles to Military Road (CR 20). Turn east and continue 3 miles to the park entrance. Drive to the interpretive center and park. The trail starts at the north end of the parking lot.

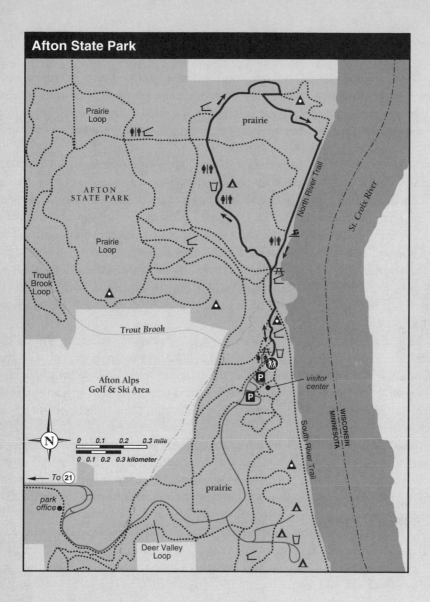

Afton State Park

If you take the trail to the far left, you'll climb steep ravines to a savannalike plateau encircled by trails. Major horseback-riding trails and hiking trails depart from this meadow, cutting back down through more ravines on the west end of the park to form a large looping network of trails.

Save those trails for another day, and instead head straight along the trail leading up to the backpackers' camping area. The trail twists uphill through stands of oaks and maples. This trail leads to some of the highest points in the northern section of the park—with a rise of more than 200 feet in the first 0.3 mile. It's a gradual ascent with a turnout observation point and rest stop that overlooks the ravine to the southwest.

Reaching the plateau, the trail levels off and opens up onto grassy corridors between islands of scrub oak and bushes. Numbered trail spurs head off perpendicular from this trail to the dozen campsites scattered throughout the area. Lying off the trail and cut into the edge of the woods, campsites are fairly well hidden and obscured from view from the main trail.

A gravel trail, supplied firewood, toilets, and water (at campsite 10) are nice amenities for campers. Remember this watering hole—it's a great place to replenish containers. In summer, the meadows can get very warm, and there is no shade on the open bluff tops. Be sure to stay well hydrated and use sunscreen.

As the trail winds through the eastern edge of this meadow, vistas of the St. Croix valley become more accessible. The trail continues east, swinging back to the river at the end of the camping area. There is a small stand of pines just before a grassy field on a short 0.3-mile loop (it's marked with a signpost). Early-morning hikers might stand a good chance of glimpsing deer, foxes, and badgers in this area.

The trail continues through a stand of cedars before coming to a good view across the river eastward into Wisconsin. This loop joins back into the main "campground" loop at a point labeled as a second watering hole on older maps. However, it's been a few seasons since this hand pump has seen any action. If you think you'll run dry before returning to the parking lot, better get your water back at campsite 10.

You'll still want to pass by this intersection, though, as there is a nice perch at the observation area right beyond the pump. Its vista features a grand view of the lower St. Croix before it joins the Mississippi River several miles downstream. This is also a good place to rest your legs before making the steady 200-foot descent back down a ravine and hitting the river trail again.

The trail is hard-packed earth (clay-loam soil) and heads right down the side of the ravine without many twists or turns. These ravines are typical of many in this part of the state. Walking through this modest understory, you'll spy tree trunks grown tall and somewhat spindly from the extra strain to reach sunlight above. Typically, these ravines have seasonal flowages running down them. In early spring, these areas can be especially muddy because of all the drainage patterns converging in them.

As you level out in the floodplain area of the river, you meet back up with the main river trail/bike corridor. Continuing on past this intersection allows you to step out onto the broad, sandy shoreline of the St. Croix. You can follow the rocky, sandy riverbank back to the lower picnic/swimming area or just spend some moments cooling off below the massive cottonwood canopies that tower over the edge of the river. During the summer, there will be a constant regatta of pleasure boats cruising back and forth along the river from bend to bend.

If you backtrack from the river, you'll hit the broad roadway of the main trail that parallels the banks about 50 feet above the river. This pathway is lined with birch and oak trees. Several openings keep the river in view to the east of the trail.

A little more than 0.5 mile south, the trail brings hikers back to the swim-ming area and the intersection with the trail that leads back up to the parking lot. The railroad-bed trail along the river continues on, extending south from the swimming area to the far southern corner of Afton State Park.

The climb back up the 85 stairs may seem a bit strenuous after all the ravine hiking, so consider an alternate route via a 180-degree switchback trail just beyond the stairway. Both take you to the top and back out to the parking lot before the visitor center.

NEARBY ACTIVITIES

Summer hikers who are as comfortable on a mountain bike as in hiking boots can bring their bikes or rent a bike next door at the Afton ski area, which doubles as a hilly mountain-bike playground in the summer. Winter snowshoe hikers can enjoy the same area for some of the best skiing around.

29   BARN BLUFF

IN BRIEF

Coming into Red Wing from the north, with the afternoon sun glowing on the sandstone walls of Barn Bluff, you'll take in a sight worthy of the 45-minute drive south of the Twin Cities. A landmark since people first trod the banks of the Mississippi River, Barn Bluff offers an invigorating ascent and spectacular views of the river valley and town below. The quick ascent via switchbacks to the base of the bluff, followed by a long stair climb to the plateau, makes this a serious urban hike.

DESCRIPTION

"The most beautiful prospect that the imagination can form." That's how 18th-century explorer Jonathan Carver described the view from Barn Bluff. Rising 343 feet above the town of Red Wing, Barn Bluff still evokes similar feelings from many. Henry David Thoreau probably agreed when he climbed it as a tourist. Stephen H. Long, the topographic engineer on an 1819 mapping expedition, no doubt found the view from Barn Bluff alluring as well.

In the local Dakota tribal legends, the big bluff was the basis for a great tale. Two tribes fought over the "ownership" of the bluff to such an extent that the Great Spirit is said

KEY AT-A-GLANCE INFORMATION

LENGTH: 1.75 miles

CONFIGURATION: Loop; random hiking once on top of bluff

DIFFICULTY: Steep; can be treacherous in winter and late spring

SCENERY: Birch- and maple-covered slopes plus an incredible 360-degree view of the Mississippi

EXPOSURE: Mostly full sun at the top; shaded woods below

TRAFFIC: Popular on bright, sunny days during summer

TRAIL SURFACE: Well worn with exposed roots and rocks; very narrow in some places; on plateau, open grasses and some worn trails network along bluff top

HIKING TIME: 1.5–2.5 hours

SEASON: Best late spring–fall

ACCESS: No fees

MAPS: Interpretive map at trailhead and online at livehealthyredwing .org/maps.htm

FACILITIES: None, although trailhead is at edge of residential and downtown districts; parking limited to narrow strip along street

SPECIAL COMMENTS: I rate this as one of the best hikes in this area due to the view and the challenging riverside access.

CONTACT: (651) 385-3655 or red-wing.org/redwingparks.html

GPS TRAILHEAD COORDINATES

Latitude   N92° 31.143'
Longitude   W44° 34.083'

Directions ———————————→

From the Twin Cities, take US 61 south from Hastings. Continue on US 61 through Red Wing to the south side of town. Barn Bluff looms ahead. Turn right at the last stoplight, and go to 5th Street. Turn left on 5th and follow it, first parallel to US 61 and then under the highway overpass, to the parking area immediately on your right. The staircase to the trailhead is on the left, just across the street.

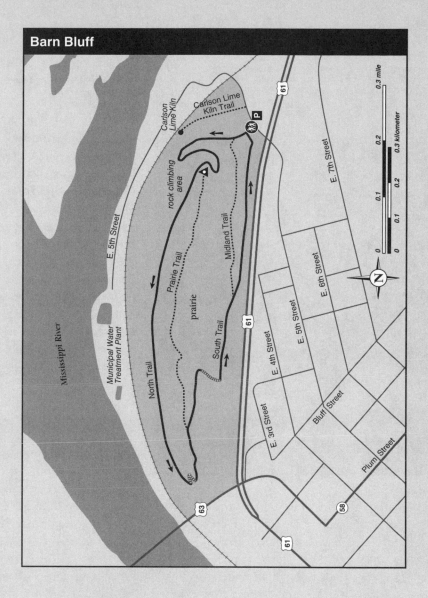

to have split the massive rock in two so each tribe could have part of it. (The other half is said to be Sugar Loaf down in Winona, about 60 miles downstream.) The French named it La Grange, which translates as "the barn." Hence its more common name, Barn Bluff.

The bluff stands as a natural demarcation of the local geologic strata in the area. Glaciers carved deep channels around some of the more resistant formations, leaving huge islands in the inland sea created when ice thawed and retreated. A stratified history of the deposits is clearly exposed in the layers that make up Barn Bluff: Franconia green sandstone only 6–8 feet above the river, St. Lawrence dolostone (blue shale) for the next 45 feet up, Jordan sandstone (layers of white-yellow stone) for another 120 feet. These combine to form Barn Bluff's Cambrian layer,

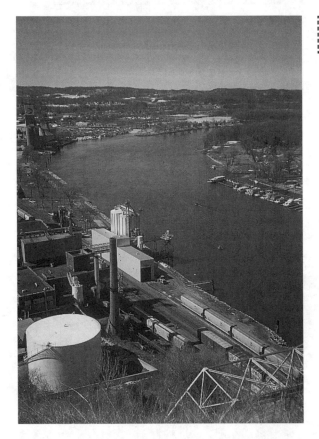

Industrial Red Wing seen from
atop Barn Bluff

dated between 500 and 540 million years old. A layer 75 feet thick of Prairie du Chien sandstone from the Ordovician period—500 to 440 million years ago—lies below the layer that caps the bluff—a relic of the Pleistocene era a mere 1.8 million to 11,000 years ago. Some of these layers are exposed via erosion nearer the start of the climb and later come into view as you ascend the bluff at just a dozen yards (in elevation) above the river.

To start this hike, park at the turnout just under the overpass for US 61. Climb the concrete staircase to the interpretive rest area to begin the actual trek around and up Barn Bluff.

I chose the path to the right. In late winter, with snow on the ground, this is a formidable path and can be very icy and unstable. However, it is the best trail to take for splendid river views, so pick your season.

The trail winds through an understory made up mostly of oaks with some maples. This is a steady uphill climb over exposed ruts, irregular rocks, and narrow pathways. It continues up the southeasternmost end of the bluff. About 150 yards up the trail, just as you get a clear view over the edge to the river below and the Izaak Walton League clubhouse, there is a stone arch outlining a tunnel into the mountain. History buffs can scout out its purpose. It may be just an old storage chamber carved into the wall. I'd question its safety and suggest you don't trespass. At this point you are nearing the base of the exposed rocky cap of the bluff and are about 75 feet above the river.

You come to an abrupt switchback that turns sharply to the left and back toward US 61. This portion of the trail becomes even steeper and narrower. It, too, is hazardous, with exposed rocks and more roots. This curving, climbing trail takes you back to the highway side of the bluff and puts you right at the base of the rocks that cap Barn Bluff. The trail turns back again toward the river and continues west along the base of the rocks for the entire length of the bluff.

The trail runs along the shoulder of relatively level ground between the bottom of the rocks and the steep descent to the river a couple hundred feet below. Railroad tracks parallel the base of the bluff, followed halfway around by a road that leads to a water-treatment facility. Beyond the road is the bank of the river.

After traversing the length of the bluff, the trail heads back around the other side of the ridge just as the Eisenhower Bridge comes into view beyond the trees. The trail shrinks here and poses a few obstacles around fallen chunks of cliff side.

At the extreme western end of the bluff is a set of concrete stairs, more than 200 in all, that make a 180-degree switchback halfway up to take hikers to the exposed cap of this great bluff. The top of the stairs yields a breathtaking view of downtown Red Wing, upriver on the Mississippi and across the Eisenhower Bridge into Wisconsin. Your prospecting imagination finally pays off when you look out over this platform at the head of those 200-plus steps.

The journey takes on a whole new hiking theme, as you can now walk casually up the slope some 30 feet more to be truly on top of the bluff. The vistas are remarkable, particularly to the north and west. A line of gnarly oaks and the whitest aspens I've ever seen grow along the northern edge of the cap.

As you reach the top of the cap and look along its entire length, there are two trails. One leads to the right; the other extends farther along the top of the cap. If you want to explore the summit, opt for the left trail and take your time; you could spend hours hiking the top. If you choose to retreat from the cap, take the trail on the right. This leads you back to the south face of the bluff for the long, gradual descent to the interpretive rest area.

The trail begins as a gradual descent and then makes a sharp turn to the right and down yet another flight of concrete stairs, a drop of about 50 feet over nine sets of six steps each. This is the alternate winter route that leads off from the left fork at the interpretive area. In late spring, this is the far safer route since its exposure to the sun makes it much less icy and snowpacked than the northern face.

Once you descend the staircase, you'll find a trail to the right, which follows a short loop to a secluded local campfire area. Also, a narrow foot trail along the base of the cliff leads back to the first long stairway to the top. This trail is less used and more dangerous than the designated routes shown on maps.

At the base of the stairs to the left is the long, gradual slope back down to the original trailhead. The trail cuts through a forested area of oaks and maples with moderate understory. This trail drops steadily for about 0.3 mile and will eventually level off as it meets up and runs parallel to US 61. A couple hundred yards farther, the path returns to the first set of stairways you took up from the parking area.

NEARBY ACTIVITIES

The town of Red Wing, with shops, restaurants, riverfronts, and historic buildings, is worth a day's visit. You aren't that far away from other hikes: Frontenac, Miesville Ravine, and Hay Creek are all to the south, less than a half hour away.

30 CANNON VALLEY TRAIL

KEY AT-A-GLANCE INFORMATION

LENGTH: 5- to 10-mile sections of 19.5-mile trail

CONFIGURATION: Out-and-back with several point-to-point options

DIFFICULTY: Mostly flat with a few gentle rises and dips throughout

SCENERY: Lush hardwood forests and bottomlands; open meadows; vistas of the river corridor; farmland

EXPOSURE: Full shade in wooded areas; open sunny fields

TRAFFIC: Predominantly bike traffic, heavier near communities at ends

TRAIL SURFACE: 8-foot-wide paved surface, with wooden bridges

HIKING TIME: 2–5 hours, depending on segments

SEASON: Year-round

ACCESS: No fee for hiking

MAPS: Online at cannonvalleytrail .com or at kiosk at Welch Station

FACILITIES: Restrooms, water, and picnic tables at Welch Station

SPECIAL COMMENTS: Parking areas are 5–9 miles apart, but there are crossings where a few cars can park off the trail. The trail has many segments you can hike, but take an out-and-back route or shuttle.

CONTACT: (507) 263-0508; Welch Station Access: (651) 258-4141

GPS TRAILHEAD COORDINATES

Latitude	N92° 44.301'
Longitude	W44° 33.784'

IN BRIEF

Typical of converted railroad beds with long straightaways and graceful curves, this trail courses through a beautiful southern Minnesota river valley. There are several points along the river where you can stop and enjoy views up, down, and across this gently flowing river (with occasional riffles).

DESCRIPTION

Like most trails developed from converted railroad beds, the Cannon Valley Trail is a long, flat corridor stretching across the countryside between two communities. In this case the countryside skirts the banks of the Cannon River as it meanders lazily between Cannon Falls on the west to Red Wing on the banks of the Mississippi River at the east end. This 19.5-mile stretch of paved trail is a bikers' highway that is also great for hiking. However, the official parking areas

----

Directions ⟶

WELCH STATION ACCESS: Take US 61 south toward Red Wing. Take CR 7 (about 1.7 miles past MN 316) to Welch Village. Continue on through village and over river for about 0.5 mile to the sign on right for Cannon Valley Trail and Hidden Valley Campground. Access station lies 50 yards ahead on left.

CANNON FALLS ACCESS: In Cannon Falls, from CR 19 go east to Bridge Street. Take Bridge Street north to Stoughton Street. At Stoughton, go right all the way to end and turn right toward softball fields beyond buildings. Trail access is on the right at front corner of parking lot.

CANNON BOTTOM ROAD ACCESS: From US 61, 1 mile south of first bridge over Cannon River, take Cannon Bottom Road for about 0.3 mile. Immediately past trail crossing, take right into parking area.

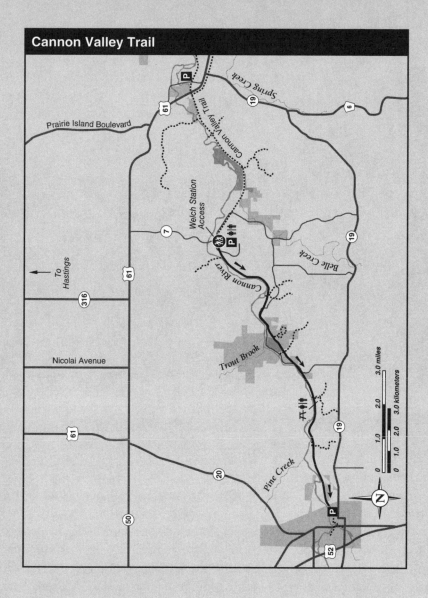

are few and far between, which means you hike out and back, have a car parked along the route, or make the full 9-plus-mile push to either end from the middle trailhead access at Welch Station.

Given those considerations, my choice section to hike is between Anderson Memorial Rest Area at Trail Run Creek about 4 miles east of Cannon Falls to the Cannon Bottom Road parking area some 5 miles east of Welch Station and 4 miles west of Red Wing. In order to enjoy this segment, one can use the parking area at Welch Station and head out in either direction for a long but gentle route with splendid views along the way.

The Welch Station Access rest area has a plethora of information. You can get trail maps, learn the geological and cultural history of the region, check out nearby

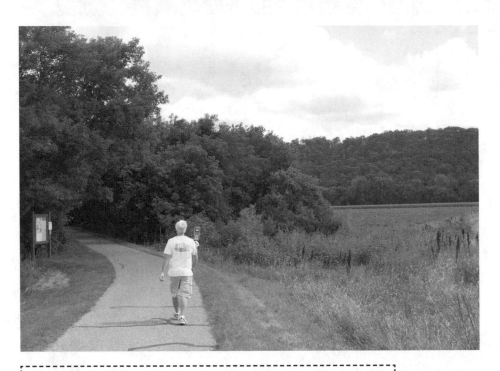

The Cannon Valley Trail follows the Cannon River through woods and along fields.

amenities, and more—all posted on the kiosk at the site. Restrooms, picnic tables, and drinking water are all in place here to make this a great staging area for users of the trail.

Heading west down this tree-lined corridor, you come upon a landmark that will be part of a series of references along the route. The 4-foot concrete obelisk on the left is a mile marker (Mile 83) for the old Chicago Great Western Railroad line that used to chug along this same route beginning in 1882. This marker told engineers the mileage from Mankato. Today there are newer mile markers, but these old, weatherworn ones remind us of the trail's railroad heritage.

The next mile of trail follows the river flanked by steep, tree-covered slopes all along the southern (left) side of the trail. Through the trees on the right are glimpses of the Hidden Valley Campground. If you don't mind unkempt, primitive campsites (even though most have electricity), you may like to camp here. The trail takes a straight course past steep slopes forested in a scattering of paper birches intermixed among the maples. You will start to catch glimpses of the river on your right. There is a bench under a basswood clump near railroad mile marker 82.

A little farther, you will come to yet another mile marker (Mile 8). This is one of the official trail markers counting the miles from Cannon Falls to the west. You are now about 2.5 miles down the trail (making this a 5-mile hike if you turn around now). Continuing on, the trail curves to the right (northerly). The understory changes as the slopes on the left pull down and back from the trail. The adjacent woods are mainly oaks, maples, and basswoods as the trail approaches and crosses a 120-foot wooden-planked bridge over a broad rock-bed wash. You can see the tops of the trees on a ridge across the river from the middle of the bridge.

As you leave the bridge behind, look down the trail and see the road crossing at about mile 3 from the start of your hike. There, a small off-road space where you could park a car offers a good end point for a short, but very representative, taste of this wonderful country trail. This is the Sand Road crossing at about mile marker 7 when measuring from the western end of the Cannon Valley Trail. Here you'll get a good view of the rural farm setting of the area. I was on this trail a few hours after sunrise and enjoyed the call of a rooster coming from the farmyard just up off the trail on the right.

The trail begins an incline as you pass a long wooden fence above a dirt road (a segment of the Sunset Trail) between you and the river. The fence is about 0.33 mile and ends around railroad mile marker 80. You are now at a second gravel-road crossing highlighted by an old-fashioned road mileage sign, a lighthearted touch of humor amid this bucolic setting. Knowing you are 7,241 miles from Tokyo may make you appreciate your shorter trek. At this point, you are also 4.6 miles from Welch Station, nearly halfway to Cannon Falls.

The trail borders a clearing—open meadows and adjacent farmland—as it passes a quaint rural homestead on the left before entering a dense tunnellike corridor of trees. The character of the trail changes slightly as exposed rocks begin to draw attention to the slopes on the left. A bit farther on, some rocks have broken off the outcrops to form a cavelike hole at the base of the trail.

The slopes open up again, and if you hike this section in the midmorning hours, you'll be treated to spears of sunlight penetrating the leafy canopy overhead. At about 4 miles from Cannon Falls (nearly 6 miles from Welch Station), a huge rock wall borders the left side of the trail. This is just before yet another wooden-planked bridge that brings you into the Anderson Memorial Rest Area.

Instead of continuing along the trail into Cannon Falls, I stopped here and hiked back to my car at Welch Station. If I were to continue into Cannon Falls, I would end up at a parking lot just down from a short spur leading off to the right from the trail. This is the western trailhead for the Cannon Valley Trail.

A convenient way to break this trail up into smaller units is to head out from the Cannon Bottom Road access parking to explore the eastern half of this trail from the Red Wing end.

For this segment, take US 61 toward Red Wing. As you approach Red Wing coming down from Minneapolis, Cannon Bottom Road, on the left, is 1 mile past the first bridge over the Cannon River before Red Wing. It drops down into the valley for about 0.5 mile to a small, gravel parking area on the right. From here you can take the trail east into the city's west edge or hike back toward Welch Station, 8 miles to the west. Heading out along the trail back toward Welch Station, you will

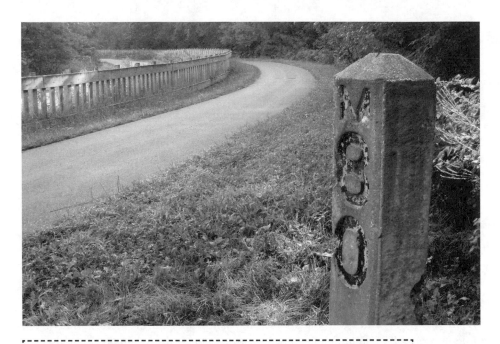

A concrete mileage marker reminds hikers of the Cannon River trail's railroad history.

soon come to a rest area right under the US 61 bridge. Several benches and bike racks make this a formal and official resting spot at the river's edge.

The trail continues along fields, through dense stands of hardwoods, and then along the edge of fields before reaching the midpoint on the trail at Welch Village. It's another great hiking route on a trail that has many segments, albeit few car-drop areas.

The Cannon Valley is rich in geological and archaeological sites, some still a mystery and as yet not thoroughly studied. The area is rich in wildlife (I saw two deer standing right on the trail), and songbirds abound. Be sure to check out the website for additional information on the fauna, flora, history, and amenities along and near this multioffering trail. It pays to study the trail map to help you decide how much you want to hike (out-and-back or one-way) on a given day. Whatever you choose, the Cannon Valley will reward you many times over.

NEARBY ACTIVITIES

You can go tubing on Cannon River at Welch Village, camp along the river at Hidden Valley (a very funky and unkempt campground), or take advantage of the shops and eateries in Cannon Falls and the historic river town of Red Wing. Miesville Ravine and Barn Bluff trails are within 10 miles of this trailhead.

COTTAGE GROVE RAVINE
REGIONAL PARK 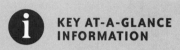 31

IN BRIEF

This moderate ravine country with solidly wooded slopes and climbs in elevation rewards you with some middistance vistas of meadows and farmland up on top. Trails make it easy to climb and descend from ravine to ridge to ravine throughout the park.

DESCRIPTION

Twenty years ago, when I was a county planner in Washington County, Cottage Grove Ravine Regional Park was one of my projects for developing the area's recreational potential. At that time the county didn't own as much land as it does now, so development was limited to the overlook parking area and the picnic area at the western edge of the lake. Now, two decades later, I am happy to report that additional land means additional areas for trail development—and what a network of trails it is!

The ravines in this park are quite impressive. Most drain into the Mississippi about 1 mile to the west and only a few miles north from where the St. Croix joins it on its way south. An interpretive map near the picnic pavilion shows the interconnecting array of trails that have been cut through the ravine and upper meadows. All trail intersections have numbered posts to make map reading virtually foolproof.

Directions ⟶

From Minneapolis or southern St. Paul, take I-494 to US 10 and US 61 south toward Hastings. Exit at CR 19 (the exit past 90th Street), and go up and over US 61 to the service road heading south. The park entrance is about 0.2 mile on left.

GPS TRAILHEAD COORDINATES

Latitude   N92° 54.012'

Longitude   W44° 48.383'

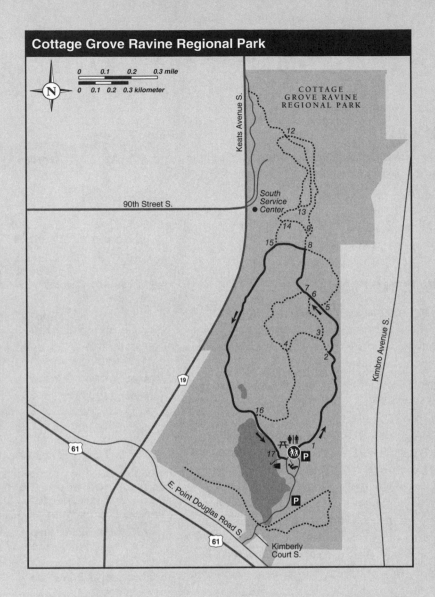

Cottage Grove Ravine Regional Park

From the parking lot, take the far right trail heading north. The path climbs casually but steadily, passing birches, maples, ashes, and other old-stand hardwoods that line the ravine feeding southward toward the lake at Cottage Grove. As you approach intersection 2, you'll see more aspens mixed in with the hardwoods.

Continue hiking straight ahead, and just beyond this intersection, after about 80 yards or so, you'll come to an open swath of grass through the woods. This is an underground utilities corridor that bisects the park and continues to its western boundary at CR 19. It's a good reference point when hiking any of the trails along either side of trail intersections 2 and 16.

The trail follows this corridor for about 0.2 mile, leading hikers through upland oaks and a few more aspens. You are above the ravines now, and, although wooded, the terrain is more even. Pass intersection 5, one of several options that offer diversity in the park. All side trails tend to join with the main trail after only 0.2 or 0.3 mile.

Continue past intersection 6 and reach intersection 7, which appears to be the highest point in the park. From here, the trails to the north wind through wooded or cleared cropland. Continue north along the main trail, leaving the cleared utility corridor behind. The trees here consist of more oaks, some cedars and pines, and more aspens, and the understory includes snowberries and sumacs. The park then opens up to meadowlike grasslands with islands of trees throughout. A line of white pines delineates one section of grasslands, while sumac, willow, and ash trees are encroaching on other open areas.

Just past the row of pines, more meadowlike areas provide longer vistas of the rolling hills and meadows to the east. Other stands of pines can be seen from this elevated area of the park. This part of Cottage Grove is similar to the neighboring parks to the east that border the St. Croix—high-meadow bluff tops with steep, tree-covered ravines cutting down toward the main drainages.

At intersection 8, turn left and follow a short but steep descent to intersection 15, which quickly brings you into ravine country. The understory is predominantly prickly ashes and sumacs, and trees typical of lower slopes and ravines again dominate.

Approximately 0.1 mile south of this intersection is the westernmost edge of the same utility corridor you crossed earlier. At this point, you are about 0.5 mile from the northwest tip of the park's main lake. From here the trail descends at a steady, unchanging rate.

Just before the trail turns sharply to the left and the lake comes into view, you'll see a well-worn but unmarked trail to the left. Take this spur trail about 40 yards to a small pond not shown on the map. Look—quietly—for ducks and more-reclusive shorebirds here in the summer.

Return to the main trail and continue on.

Some maps show a trail completely around the lake in the basin of Cottage Grove Ravine Regional Park. I saw no evidence of the trail around the far side of the lake. I could find no access trail from the extreme northwest end, either. Stick to the north side of the lake for a glimpse of the other shoreline. A good set of binoculars will keep you from missing any scenery or critters.

The trail follows the lake for about 0.2 mile before returning to the parking and picnic area.

NEARBY ACTIVITIES

Several parks and hiking areas are scattered along the US 61 corridor, both to the north and to the south of Cottage Grove Ravine. US 10 leads south to Point Douglas Park at the confluence of the Mississippi and St. Croix rivers. Right across the river is Prescott, Wisconsin.

32 FRONTENAC STATE PARK,
Bluffside Trail

KEY AT-A-GLANCE INFORMATION

LENGTH: 2.5 miles

CONFIGURATION: Short loop coupled with an elongated loop

DIFFICULTY: Difficult along 400-foot bluffs with steep ravines and intersecting trails; switchbacks help

SCENERY: Impressive valleys, overlooks, mature stands of oak and maple, open meadow atop bluffs

EXPOSURE: Exposed meadows atop bluff; dense canopies in ravines

TRAFFIC: A park known well by locals, but a mystery to many

TRAIL SURFACE: Grassy lanes to narrow trails cut into the slopes; slippery in spots when wet

HIKING TIME: 1.5–2.5 hours

SEASON: Year-round, but steep trails are best in summer

ACCESS: Minnesota State Park fee system: $5 daily, $25 annual permit, $12 annual permit for disabled individuals

MAPS: At park or at www.dnr.state.mn.us/state_parks/frontenac

FACILITIES: Campsites, restrooms, showers, and more

SPECIAL COMMENTS: Great hiking with incredible scenery and history

CONTACT: (651) 345-3401

GPS TRAILHEAD COORDINATES

Latitude   N92° 20.172'

Longitude   W44° 32.095'

IN BRIEF

One of my favorite parks, Frontenac offers exceptional trails along some of the steepest bluffs in the area. (This route can be made into an out-and-back if the bluff-line hike proves too difficult.) With more geological and cultural history than parks three times its size, Frontenac State Park is truly a hidden treasure, well worth the drive south of the Cities.

DESCRIPTION

This is one of those parks with such a fantastic history that you are compelled to learn about it before you take to the trails. Knowing an area's geological beginnings and the cast of players who helped establish the region's history adds to the personality of any site, and this one in particular.

Hundreds of millions of years ago, Minnesota was covered by a shallow sea. Sediment accumulated at its bottom and slowly changed into rock. That rock is now visible as the bluffs of the Mississippi River. In glacial times a gigantic river, called the River Warren, was fed from glacial runoff. It carved the giant valleys through which many of Minnesota's rivers now flow. At its peak, most of Frontenac was underwater—except for the park's bluff.

In more recent history, archeological digs at Frontenac in 1976 uncovered artifacts from the Hopewellian culture dating from 400 BC to AD 300. Some of these sites were

----

Directions ———————————→

From the Twin Cities, take US 61 south. Frontenac is 10 miles south of Red Wing. Turn left (east) on CR 2, and go about 1 mile. Entrance is on left. Drive to end of road and park.

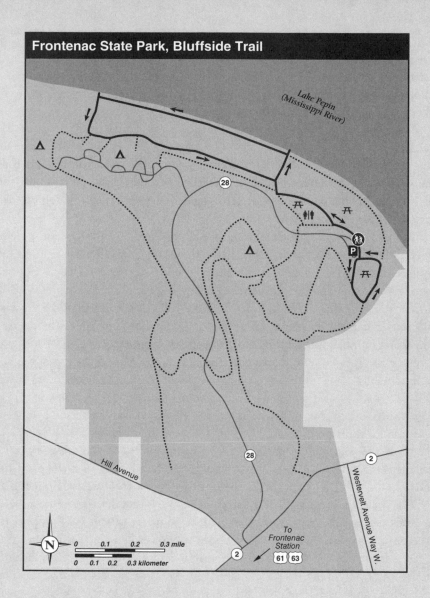

Lake Pepin
(Mississippi River)

To
Frontenac
Station

Hill Avenue

Westervelt Avenue Way W.

0   0.1   0.2   0.3 mile

0   0.1   0.2   0.3 kilometer

burial grounds; other findings indicate that the tribes lived in the area as well.

Dakota and Fox Native Americans later settled in this valley, followed by French explorers who might have actually built the first church in Minnesota here. The famous French missionary Father Louis Hennepin led the first European exploration to this area of the Mississippi River in 1680.

In 1727, an expedition left Montreal to set up a post in this area to launch further exploration westward in search of a route to the Pacific Ocean. The French-Indian War caused these settlements to be abandoned until the mid-1800s, when the first permanent pioneers settled.

By the 1870s, Frontenac was enjoying status as a premier tourist destination, a resort town drawing visitors on riverboats from as far downriver as New Orleans. Looking out over the valley today, with views of trains along the river, small towns and farmsteads, and forested bluffs, you can truly sense the spirit of the area.

A number of trailheads leave from various points along the parking lot. This hike starts out with the short but intense interpretive trail loop off the eastern end of the main picnic area parking lot. Having a map handy at the onset is advisable because of the trail options available. Whether you tackle the full extent of the Bluffside Trail or the much less strenuous meadow network of trails, you owe it to yourself to take this loop first.

The interpretive trail packs the essence of the entire park into a short, dense, looped trail. Trailheads are not always marked, but the available maps are accurate. The start of the trail is well marked and beckons hikers with a groomed, 3-foot-wide grassy lane through aspens and oaks. Several trails extend off this pathway to the right, including an out-and-back spur about 0.1-mile long, marked as the Observation Point Trail, that heads out from the parking lot trailhead to a beautiful overlook of the valleys to the south and the old town site of Frontenac.

Back on the main interpretive trail, the path descends over the top of the bluff line and literally down into the geological history of the park. The bluff now behind you used to be the only point of land in an inland sea that covered all of what is now the great Mississippi Valley. With their steep, 400-foot embankment still below you, the sandstone bluffs provide a narrow line for this path to follow.

Along the way, mature paper birches, sugar maples, and cottonwoods guard the banks. A moderate understory is below you, and a wall of worn sandstone stands like a fortress on your left—some of this exposed rock reaches 30 feet high.

This area is known as Garrard's Bluff, after the founder of Frontenac, General Israel Garrard. Riverboat pilots named the same area Point-No-Point because of the optical illusion that it was a true point of land when viewed from upriver.

Evidence of quarry activity can be found in a few of the iron rings still solidly fastened into the ground near the quarry site. Many architects favored this high-quality rock, and the Cathedral of St. John the Divine, in New York City, is made of Frontenac limestone from this quarry. Imagine the restraints needed to lower massive blocks of limestone down the steep 400-foot embankment to waiting barges on the river below.

At about this point, the trail intersects with a steep trail dropping to the right and away from the base of the bluffs to the riverbanks below. Take this trail and then go left at the river. Continue for another 1.1 miles before heading back up to the top of the bluff. Here the Mississippi River broadens into the start of Lake Pepin. By the time the river reaches Lake City, about 5 miles to the south, it's more than 3 miles wide.

This area along the river is renowned for bird-watching. Both the river area and the upper bluffs are visited by passing species during spring migration. The hardwoods in the bottomlands create a perfect nesting habitat for the prothonotary warbler. Watch along the river during spring and fall migration for sanderlings and ruddy turnstones, shorebirds that travel between South America and the Arctic each year. Bring your bird book and binoculars, as more than 200 species have been sighted throughout the park.

The segment climbing back up toward the top of the bluff measures 0.3 mile and leads up to a T intersection at the base of the bluff. At the T, there is a short spur to the left. This leads to a distinctive natural landmark—a huge rock with a hole in it positioned close to the edge of the bluff. Called In-Yan-Teopa in the language of the local Native Americans, this massive rock outcrop may have had some religious significance.

A short trail spur leading back from the rock returns you to the bluff trail. Turn left, which brings you to the observation platform above In-Yan-Teopa. From the observation platform, you can either continue along the base of the rocky bluff, or take the trail straight back from the observation deck that leads up to the edge of the campground, where a second trail follows along the top of the bluff— and also leads back to the main parking lot.

However, stay on the lower of the two trails. As you advance along the base of the rocky ledge, you will see two short spurs to the right that head up to the campgrounds. Stay on the main trail for the next 0.5 mile; then you will come to an intersection with a third trail. This trail crosses the bluff trail from its trailhead at the picnic area atop the bluff on its way down to the river. If you take the right fork at this intersection, you just parallel the trail you are on, as they both continue for 0.2 mile back to the steep switchback staircase at the end of the interpretive loop that will take you up to the top of the bluff and back to the parking lot at the picnic area.

At the top of the switchbacks, another observation deck provides fantastic views of the Mississippi River Valley. The trail rejoins the picnic area and the parking lot at the opposite end of the interpretive loop near where you started.

This hike only scratches the surface of the trails available here. Additional hiking opportunities exist south of the picnic area. Those trails wind across and along upland meadows all along the bluff tops, after which they again drop down into the ravines on the back side of the river bluffs. The northwest loops of the trails cut through the walk-in camping area and create a network of trails along the grassy meadows between the ravines. A 1.5-mile loop descends one ravine, follows the park road, and then climbs back up another ravine to the bluff-top meadows along the upper road system and the developed area of the park.

NEARBY ACTIVITIES

I'd have a hard time leaving this park, but a trip to old-town Frontenac is worth a visit. If you are a golfer, one of the prettiest and hilliest courses in the area is right across the road at Frontenac Golf Course; for tee times, call (651) 388-5826 or (800) 488-5826. The course has incredible vistas on top of the bluffs even higher than those at Frontenac State Park.

33 LEBANON HILLS REGIONAL PARK,
Holland/Jensen Lakes Loop

KEY AT-A-GLANCE INFORMATION

LENGTH: 2.6 miles

CONFIGURATION: Balloon

DIFFICULTY: Easy to moderate; numerous small changes in elevation

SCENERY: Peaceful and picturesque, from rolling hills to quiet lakes

EXPOSURE: Wooded, shady areas evenly mixed with open meadows

TRAFFIC: Very popular, particularly with joggers

TRAIL SURFACE: Wide, compacted grass trails; some earthen paths

HIKING TIME: 1.5 hours

SEASON: Year-round; hunting is briefly allowed in fall; many trails are open for cross-country skiing

ACCESS: No fees

MAPS: Dakota County Parks map at the visitor center and online at tinyurl.com/lebanonhillspark

FACILITIES: Parking, picnic shelter, swimming beach, playground, canoe trail, restrooms at trailhead, campground, potable water nearby

SPECIAL COMMENTS: Surrounded by town houses, strip malls, and freeways, this park sees heavy use yet maintains its country character.

CONTACT: (952) 891-7000

GPS TRAILHEAD COORDINATES

Latitude   N93° 8.704'

Longitude   W44° 47.389'

IN BRIEF

Located in the heart of the suburbs south of Minneapolis, Lebanon Hills is one of the more diverse parks in the Dakota County system. There are more than a dozen lakes scattered throughout rolling hills with clusters of oaks and maples and open pockets of meadows and marshes. One of the prettiest lakes in the region—unnamed no less—greets hikers deep within the park.

DESCRIPTION

Like so many other suburban parks that sit in the middle of residential suburban sprawl, Lebanon Hills quickly lures the visitor into the heart of the park and away from any reminders of that fringe of development. The Holland/Jensen Lakes trail leads the hiker away from the big houses skirting the boundary of the park and into hilly terrain covered in oaks and meadows, sprinkled with ponds and lakes.

Dropping down from the parking lot, take the spur trail leading along the west side of Holland Lake toward a network of trails that allow you to select from several loop options. Most will lead back to this short 0.25-mile segment and a brief, repeated journey up this same trail spur. In the spring, or after a good rain, expect this first section around

Directions

From Minneapolis, drive south on Cedar Avenue/MN 77 to Cliff Road (Exit 4A). From St. Paul, drive south on I-35 East to Cliff Road (Exit 93); turn left (east) and drive past Pilot Knob Road to the Holland Lake entrance on the right. The trailhead is at the parking lot's far right corner.

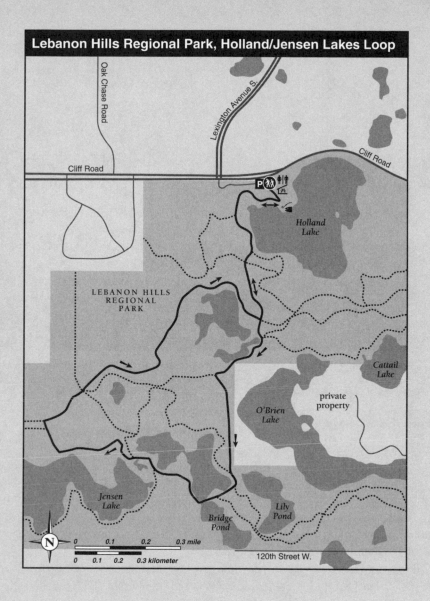

Holland Lake to be a bit wet. The trail winds through a fairly thick growth of aspen, birch, wild cherry, and buckthorn before encountering one of the many hills of Lebanon. Continuing through a stand of aspen, the trail soon takes hikers to an open meadow and the first of many trail intersections (all fairly well marked, but get a map at the trailhead parking lot). Each map trail marker has a "you are here" indicator that corresponds to the trail map. Continue straight ahead.

Less than 0.25 mile into the park, this trail winds its way through several species of oak that border a meadow at the southwest end of the lake. Out of the woods south of Holland Lake, the country transitions into a series of gently rolling hills. The trail is lined with sumacs, and young oaks pop up intermittently

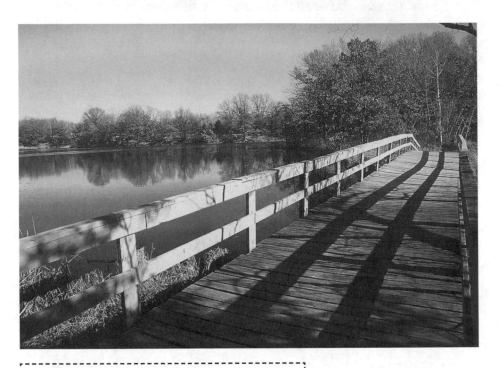

A wooden bridge links trails at Lebanon Hills Regional Park.

across the grassy fields. I was here in late fall but would expect to see a spring profusion of wildflowers common to the upland meadows of central Minnesota.

Numerous ponds—all nameless—pocket the area's recesses, adding to a pleasant country setting of rolling countryside, islands of hardwood trees, and a patchwork quilt of prairielike meadows.

Hike past another trail on your left, and as you approach the northwest corner of O'Brien Lake you'll come upon a covered picnic table and your first good glimpse of O'Brien. Stay on the trails here because most of the property around this lake is private.

You'll share the trails with joggers. The wide pathway and gently undulating terrain probably provide a good workout for runners—as they do for faster-paced hikers. After a good snowfall, you're sure to see cross-country skiers as well.

Continuing south along the western edge of the lake, the trail becomes wide and rutted—more road than trail. Just past the picnic table and a trail junction, about 200 yards farther south, a nesting platform for ospreys and other raptors has been erected atop a tall pole on the left. Approach it slowly and quietly, and you may be rewarded with a glimpse of local raptor residents.

Few sections of this trail maintain any one characteristic for very long. This rutted roadway soon opens onto yet another meadow with a surface that appears to have been recently scoured by a ground fire. This provides a good

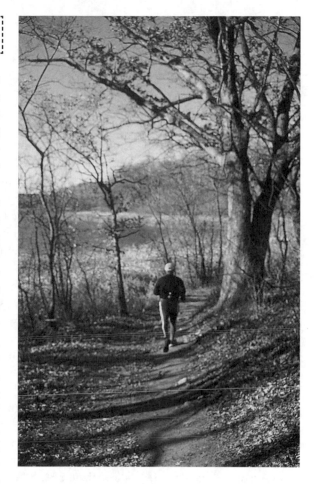

A jogger on Lebanon Hills' earthen trails

field demonstration of the positive benefits of brush fires, especially if you know what was growing here before and what successions occur as new growth emerges.

Several horse trails intertwine throughout the park, and intersections with the hiking trail are common. Personally, I try to stay away from the trails that share usage. Horse trails get ground into a very deep yet fine dust that can be tiring to walk on for any distance. Also, I have yet to experience a quiet walk when riders are present. I guess horseback riding and loud talking go hand in hand. These horse trails are pretty obvious, but are usually marked as well.

A little more than a mile along this trail on the right is a beautiful country lake surrounded by oaks and birches that blanket its steep banks. I imagine that it's beautiful in the summer because it is absolutely gorgeous in the fall. Golds, oranges, and reds are speckled throughout the trees that line the lake's banks. A shallow bay on the far side creates an opening in the shoreline, and the marshy area beyond adds a smattering of cattails to the scene. This unnamed lake is on the Jensen Lake chain.

The trail cuts deeply into the steep banks along the southeastern edge of the lake. Stately birch trees line the southern shoreline. This lake feeds into yet another at the extreme southern end. A picturesque footbridge provides a dry crossing and a dual vantage point for looking back over the first lake or southeast along the canoe route. Just before the footbridge, a small knoll with a picnic table furnishes a handy resting place for hikers and paddlers alike.

The pathway becomes more serpentine as it continues north around the western edge of this lake. Oak trees line the pockets of clearings to the west.

Less than 0.25 mile farther, Jensen Lake comes into view. Several trail inter-sections offer options should you want to extend your hike. The first one to the left (south) winds around the southern end of Jensen Lake to a T junction. From there you can continue around the entire lake to the right (for an additional 2.2 miles) or cut back to the left and toward the other parking lot and playground.

This hike stays to the right and continues along the northern shore, then loops back toward Holland Lake. The route leads past some development but will eventually get you back to the hiking trails or a short segment of one of the horse trails. The area seems especially alive with birds, so expect to see quite a few varieties in the summer. During my visit in late fall, chickadees, downy wood-peckers, and scores of cedar waxwings dominated a small section of woods just north of the trail junction that leads away from the lake.

Shortly after leaving the lake, the narrow trail intersects a road. To the right is a private residence; to the left the road leads to another parking area. A narrow pathway, straight ahead across the road, heads up through the understory. Take this trail. It breaks out onto a wider horse trail (the spot where you'd end up if you looped around Jensen Lake). Following the horse path enables you to make a loop back to the spur leading to the parking lot without a lot of backtracking.

This stretch of the trail is quite sandy in places. It's easier to walk on the edges of such trails—and probably safer. This wide section goes for about 0.3 mile through mature stands of oaks. The trail takes you back along the opposite side of the picturesque but nameless lake encountered earlier, before cutting back into the woods. Eventually you'll return to the spur that led you down from the parking lot. As you come to the end of the lake, remember to take the second trail, not the first. The second one, about 30–40 yards farther, is the correct one. It climbs back up to the park entrance where the trailhead started.

A word of caution: If you are planning a hike through Lebanon Hills in the fall, check the posted signs explaining the limited deer hunting that is allowed in this park. Typically these hunting times are restricted to a few short periods dur-ing the week, from early morning until noon.

NEARBY ACTIVITIES

The Minnesota Zoo, a few blocks away, has paved trails tying all the outside viewing areas together. Also at the zoo is an IMAX theater, which showcases wonderful programming throughout the year.

MIESVILLE RAVINE PARK RESERVE 34

IN BRIEF

One of the enjoyable attractions at this park is the drive down into it, which resembles a trip into Sleepy Hollow. Basic yet unique, it's a small park with two simple trails: one along the ravine and one along the river.

DESCRIPTION

As the county road leading into the park starts to drop down into the valley, you begin to sense that Miesville Ravine is going to be a bit rough, and totally quaint. This hike begins at the end of the north parking lot. There, a mowed, grassy corridor cuts through the thick brush understory and past tall cottonwoods lining the floor of the ravine. It follows Trout Brook for its entire length of just more than 1.5 miles.

The first 0.5 mile of the trail meanders through the large trees and gradually works its way toward the steep slopes of the ravine that line both sides of the small valley.

As you approach the stands of birches and maples, take the main trail, which splits off to the right before reconnecting to the side trail after 0.17 mile. There is a washout from the creek that could be quite muddy during high water or after a good rain. This part of the trail

----

Directions ⟶

From the Twin Cities, drive south on US 52 to Hampton. Go east on CR 50 about 9 miles to CR 91 in Miesville. Turn right, and go south on CR 91 for 1.7 miles to the intersection with 280th Street. Go left (east) on 280th Street 1.4 miles to the park entrance. Alternately, go south on US 61 to CR 50; then go east to Miesville, following the above directions south from Miesville.

ℹ KEY AT-A-GLANCE INFORMATION

LENGTH: 3.4 miles total (north trail, 1.6 miles; south trail, 1.8 miles)

CONFIGURATION: North trail is out-and-back with two short loops; south trail is loop with two return options.

DIFFICULTY: Easy and mostly level, with a gradual elevation rise on the long loop on the south trail

SCENERY: Mature stands of hardwoods and conifers; unobstructed views of Cannon River

EXPOSURE: Mostly shaded on north trail; exposed to full sun on the south trail along the river

TRAFFIC: Most activity occurs on the river; the north trail is less crowded

TRAIL SURFACE: Grassy lanes, earthen hard pack with a few wooden walkways; can be muddy in sections

HIKING TIME: 1.5–2 hours

SEASON: Year-round

ACCESS: No fees

MAPS: Available at parking lot information board or at tinyurl.com /miesville

SPECIAL COMMENTS: Although you may not happen upon this park, it's worth the effort to find. This is the backcountry at its best—narrow roads, steep ravines, dense woods, and a river.

CONTACT: (952) 891-7000

GPS TRAILHEAD COORDINATES

Latitude   N92° 48.177'
Longitude   W44° 32.596'

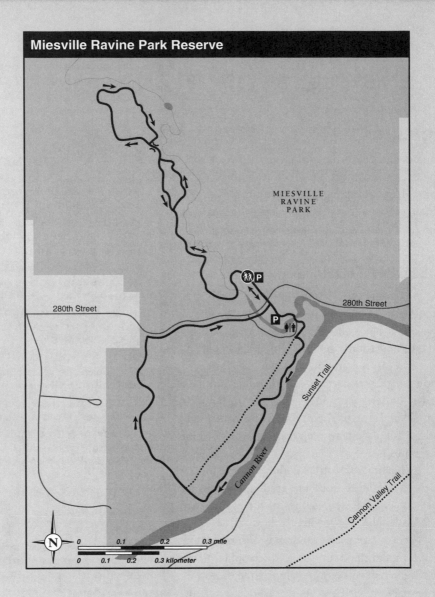

MIESVILLE
RAVINE
PARK

280th Street

280th Street

Sunset Trail

Cannon River

Cannon Valley Trail

N

0   0.1   0.2   0.3 mile

0   0.1   0.2   0.3 kilometer

winds through a dense growth of grasses, wildflowers, willows, and ashes. The vegetation is thick here, so it would be hard to get off the trail in this short section. This stretch of the trail should explode with color in May thanks to all the wildflowers in bloom. Big willow trees and mature box elders provide the canopy overhead.

Continuing on, the trail joins back into the main path for another 80 yards to arrive at yet another intersection. This is the start of an enclosed 0.46-mile loop that encircles the marshy area ahead. A wooden walkway assures dry passage over the trail at this point.

The park is home to beavers, raccoons, deer, wood ducks, ruffed grouse, and wild turkeys, so be on the watch. The trail turns back down the ravine halfway along the loop and continues through more maples and ashes. Signs of deer abound in this part of the park. As in the rest of this northern section, the pathway stays level. That means you can expect soggy trails after rains.

In the area around the wooden footbridge, you will see green, segmented, tubular plants about 2 feet tall. These are horsetails, also called Indian scrub brush because their stems contain silica. A handful of the stems, when crushed, can be used as a scouring pad in camp.

Another plant worth mentioning, found in this and other parks, is the prickly ash tree. From a distance it appears to be nothing more than a sapling of common green ash. But upon closer inspection, you can see roselike thorns all along its slender main trunk. It looks innocent until you pass too closely and feel its needle-like thorns.

Once you cross the footbridge, you are back on the main trail. It continues along the route you took down, but stay to the right and you will pick up the 0.14-mile segment you passed earlier (when you took its 0.17-mile twin). The parking lot is about 0.4 mile farther.

The southern half of the trail system continues across the road to another parking lot. This leads over a bridge to a staging area for a local outfitter's canoe trips. The Cannon River forms the southern border of Miesville Ravine Park Reserve, and the first 0.5 mile of trail follows the river along its bank. During the summer, there will be steady but lazy river traffic in the form of canoes and kayaks.

This trail is a broad lane of mowed grass. Stately oaks, of the gnarly burr oak variety, stand like sentries between the path and the river. There are several areas where you have good, open vistas of the river and can make your way down to the water's edge.

At one of these spots, you will see a rocky sandbar edging the channel. Immediately across from this area on the trail are wild plum trees. In September, their fruit is quite sweet and juicy.

After about 0.5 mile, the trail makes a 90-degree turn back into the woods. Take another right turn and you can loop back to the parking lot on a straight, level trail. However, if you keep going straight past this intersection, away from the river, you can take the long way back: another 0.3 mile of hiking.

Go for it! This trail passes the remains of an old building and continues its way back up one of the ravines that cut down to the river. As you climb up along the edge of the ravine, you'll pass through stands of birch and basswood. When you hit the dirt road, turn to the right (east) and enjoy the casual 0.4-mile walk back down the country road to the parking lot.

NEARBY ACTIVITIES

Along the road and in the park, there is good bird-watching. Be on the lookout for goldfinches, cedar waxwings, and indigo buntings. The staging area for canoes is a popular put-in spot for paddlers heading downstream a short distance to Welch Village. The midpoint access to the Cannon Valley Trail is located about 0.5 mile south of Welch Village.

35 NERSTRAND-BIG WOODS STATE PARK,
Big Woods Trail

KEY AT-A-GLANCE INFORMATION

LENGTH: 3.1 miles

CONFIGURATION: Two stacked loops

DIFFICULTY: Easy to moderate; fall leaf litter hides rocks and roots

SCENERY: Stately trees and an open understory; small waterfall in a grotto setting along trail

EXPOSURE: Mostly shade under the full canopy of the towering trees

TRAFFIC: Several places to get lost in this park; very peaceful

TRAIL SURFACE: Mostly grasses, earthen; uneven in many places

HIKING TIME: 2–2.5 hours average

SEASON: Year-round; good ski/ snowshoe trails in winter

ACCESS: Minnesota State Park fee system: $5 daily, $25 annual permit, $12 annual permit for disabled individuals

MAPS: Available at park headquarters or at www.dnr.state.mn.us /state_parks/nerstrand_big_woods

FACILITIES: Visitor center with water, restrooms, showers in summer; campground with electric sites

SPECIAL COMMENTS: Away from the freeways; surrounded by farm country and quite special woods

CONTACT: (507) 333-4840

GPS TRAILHEAD COORDINATES

Latitude   N93° 6.754'

Longitude   W44° 20.636'

IN BRIEF

Big woods, incredible fall colors, a rich geological history represented by a waterfall—all of these assets are offered on easy to moderate trails through stands of woods with ever-changing character. It's also the only place in the state to see the dwarf trout lily bloom in the spring.

DESCRIPTION

You have to know the human history of this park to fully appreciate these big woods. What remains is part of a presettlement hardwood forest that covered more than 5,000 acres hundreds of years ago. When pioneers settled here in the mid-1800s, they had the foresight to set up a small series of wooded lots that would remain unlogged. Theirs was a conservation effort based on utility—they wanted to make sure they had a sustainable supply of firewood as the woodlands fell to the clearing ax for farmland. These plots were marked out in what is now the center of Nerstrand–Big Woods State Park. Created in the 1940s, this park preserved 1,280 acres of those wooded lots.

By happenstance I hiked this trail in the fall. It was a crisp, clear day and I had camped in the park, in the primitive group camp area. I left my tent behind and headed for the trail at the end of the parking lot. The resulting hike heads into the northern section of the Big Woods, crossing Prairie Creek and connecting with a network of hiking-only trails.

Directions

Head south on I-35 to MN 19 East, and go left into Northfield. Turn right (south) on MN 3, then left (east) on MN 246. Turn right to stay on MN 246 at CR 81. Go right on CR 40 to the park entrance.

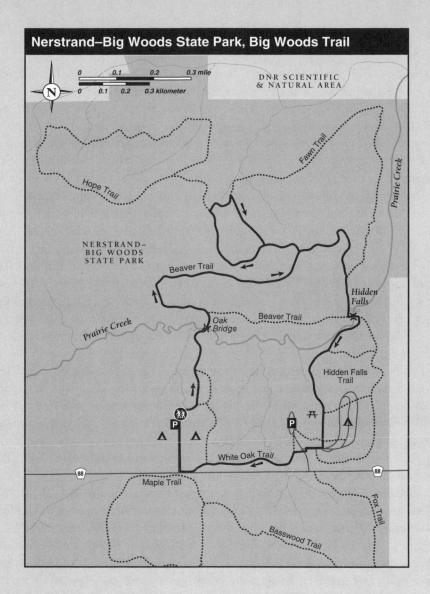

DNR SCIENTIFIC
& NATURAL AREA

Fawn Trail

Prairie Creek

Hope Trail

NERSTRAND–
BIG WOODS
STATE PARK

Beaver Trail

Hidden
Falls

Oak
Bridge

Beaver Trail

Prairie Creek

Hidden Falls
Trail

White Oak Trail

Maple Trail

Fox Trail

Basswood Trail

You immediately sense the woodsy feel of the park from the mature stands of trees and lush undergrowth along the trail that leads down to the creek. At 0.4 mile, the trail bottoms out at Prairie Creek. These are wooded lowlands typical of creek beds in the area. Oak Bridge crosses the creek here, and hikers in the mood for a shorter trip can head to the right along the Beaver Trail for 0.4 mile to Hidden Falls. But you don't want to cut the hike short, do you? The longer trek through more impressive stands and elevation changes moves back up the other side of the shallow creek valley along the White Oak Trail.

The trail climbs gradually back up to the ridge above the creek. The path is wide and easy to walk. The woods rise around you, and a dense understory right to the edge of the trail guides you along under a spreading canopy of sugar maples, basswoods, ironwoods, elms, ashes, and oaks. The White Oak Trail connects to the Hope Trail turnoff at 0.4 mile from the Beaver Trail intersection.

This trail heads back west, like a switchback of the trail below, and enters into one of my favorite areas in the park. Here, with no understory beneath a dense stand of younger maples, you walk a pathway between the golden maple leaves still clinging to the trees and those spread out as a thick, 6-inch-deep carpet across the forest floor. This beautiful glen sits in a shallow depression surrounded by the rest of the woodlands. It's one of many short segments of the trails in this park that have their own unique character. Equally impressive in the summer under a full sun, this section was likewise quite memorable in midfall.

The Hope Trail section continues for 0.3 mile before intersecting with a short trail that cuts back into the woods. If you want to tack on an additional 1.2 miles to your hike, the Hope Trail continues on and climbs upward to some grassy fields just west of the big woods. It eventually circles back down to connect to the far end of this same short segment.

Take the shortcut, and then turn right to follow the brief 0.1-mile leg down to yet another junction. This time you have of the option of hanging to the left and following the upper sections of the Fawn Trail, a 1-mile loop that winds through the northeast corner of the park, finally emerging about 0.1 mile north of Hidden Falls. If you keep to the right and continue heading southeast, Fawn Trail continues down for 0.2 mile to a section of the Hope Trail loop taken earlier. It also leads on for another 0.1 mile to the White Oak Trail's eastern 0.3-mile leg before reaching a T intersection with the eastern end of the Beaver Trail. Take a left, cross the creek, and the falls are just ahead.

Prairie Creek reveals the heart of the forest floor at Hidden Falls. In geological terms, the park sits on two nearly horizontal layers. The top is a 150-foot-thick layer of glacial drift. That layer sits on a layer of Platteville limestone. Many of the riverbanks in this region have revealed outcrops of this same limestone. The claylike material visible throughout the park is this glacial drift. Hidden Falls is the only place in the park where the limestone is revealed—exposed by the cutting action of the creek through the drift. There are also sections along the bottom of the creek where the straw-yellow limestone is likewise uncovered.

The limestone has a much longer history. It was the floor of a sea nearly 500 million years ago during the Ordovician period. During the last few ice ages, much of this part of Minnesota was forever etched by the runoff from remnants of melting ice. Prairie Creek's valley is a prime example of land sculpted in that era.

The area surrounding the falls, which consists of a series of exposed rock and low shelves of rock, would be a great place to relax on a hot day. Because it is only about 0.3 mile from the main campground, this is probably one of the most visited spots in the park.

The trail to the camp climbs a moderate grade through a thin stand of oak trees. This lies along the eastern boundary to the park. The open meadow on the left may be what this entire area would have looked like had the early settlers not protected the big woods as they did.

The trail connects with the end of a campground loop and heads toward the entrance to the park. I chose this route so I could walk the last 0.4 mile along the country road that bisects the park. At Hidden Falls Trail, you could take the Beaver Trail back to the intersection with the trail from the group camp. It's the same distance, but the Beaver Trail traces the creek along its course above Hidden Falls.

Hiking this trail in the spring will reward hikers with a variety of wildflowers including hepatica, Dutchman's-breeches, bloodroot, young fern heads, and the dwarf trout lily (found only in this park). There are lots of birds in the park, too, including blue-winged and cerulean warblers, tufted titmice, and blue-gray gnat-catchers. Make sure food and cooking items are secure in your camp, as many bold raccoons live in the campgrounds.

NEARBY ACTIVITIES

A working dairy farm, Big Woods Dairy is a special project run by a family that tends 50 dairy cattle on 80 acres using a rotational grazing system. Plans are to open the dairy farm one day each year for visitors.

36 SPRING LAKE PARK RESERVE, Schaar's Bluff Trail

KEY AT-A-GLANCE INFORMATION

LENGTH: 2.9 miles

CONFIGURATION: Two loops

DIFFICULTY: Easy; mostly level with a few gradual slopes; side trails require a little more careful footing.

SCENERY: Magnificent views of Spring Lake on the Mississippi and the river valley; expansive meadows rich in summer wildflowers

EXPOSURE: Wooded areas quite dense along bluff; full exposure on trails through open meadows

TRAFFIC: Once trail levels in public area, there are long, uncrowded stretches.

TRAIL SURFACE: Mostly wide, 8-foot lanes with a few narrow game trail spurs, particularly on northern loop

HIKING TIME: 1.25–2 hours

SEASON: Year-round; some trails groomed for cross-country skiing

ACCESS: $7 during summer months; $6 the rest of the year

MAPS: At park headquarters or at tinyurl.com/springlakereserve

FACILITIES: Fully developed day-use park with picnic area, restrooms, drinking water, playground

SPECIAL COMMENTS: Take the time to enjoy the short spur trails.

CONTACT: (952) 891-7000

GPS TRAILHEAD COORDINATES

Latitude   N92° 56.136'

Longitude   W44° 46.052'

IN BRIEF

Truly a park that feels like northern Minnesota in its scenic bluff-line trails and woodlands, Spring Lake Park Reserve has incredible vistas of the Mississippi River—all captured along the Schaar's Bluff Trail.

DESCRIPTION

As well groomed and nicely developed as this park unit is, I was surprised to find such rustic, natural trail segments. Spring Lake Park Reserve has been called the "hidden jewel" of the Upper Mississippi. Like so many other hikes along the Mississippi corridor, the Schaar's Bluff trail system showcases the scenic bluff area of the Mississippi in a widening of the river called Spring Lake. The park is only a few miles upstream from the confluence of the St. Croix River.

Starting at the parking lot, take the trail that heads east (right) into the woods at the edge of the grassy extensions of the picnic and play areas. In fact, the first 0.5 mile of this trail appears to have been laid out by someone who couldn't decide whether to walk through the woods or along the open spaces. The trail does both. It's a wide, mowed avenue through basswoods, oaks, and ashes. The trail snakes in and out of these woods twice before finally turning toward

Directions

From Minneapolis/St. Paul, take US 52 south to MN 55. Turn left (east) toward Hastings. Drive 4.5 miles to CR 42; then turn left and go 1.8 miles to Idell Avenue. Take another left, and follow this road 1 mile to park entrance. Turn right into park, and drive to parking lot at end of road.

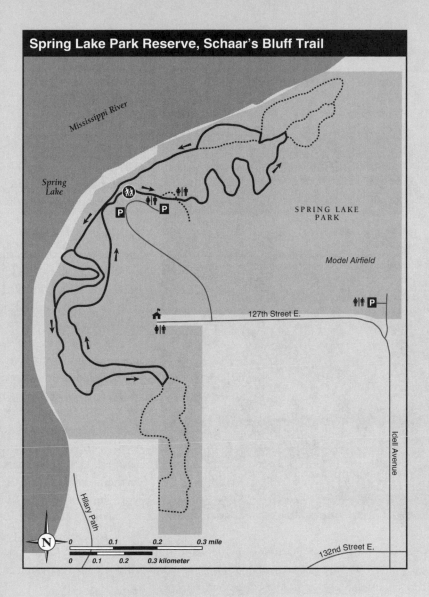

Mississippi River

Spring
Lake

SPRING LAKE
PARK

Model Airfield

127th Street E.

Idell Avenue

Hillary Path

132nd Street E.

N

0   0.1   0.2   0.3 mile

0   0.1   0.2   0.3 kilometer

the top of the bluffs high above the river. The first part of the trail could be muddy after rains or during the spring thaw. There are now red maples and red oaks mixed in with the other hardwoods.

At 0.57 mile from the trailhead, the path intersects one of two short spur trails. If you go right and take the 0.3-mile loop through the woods, it will bring you back to the same intersection. This loop also connects to another 0.29-mile loop that draws you even closer to the bluff line before returning to the trail. These trails are unnamed but are well marked on the map, with distances listed for each segment.

If you save these optional loops for another day, continue past the first intersection and go a short distance (about 80 yards) to the next one. This is the

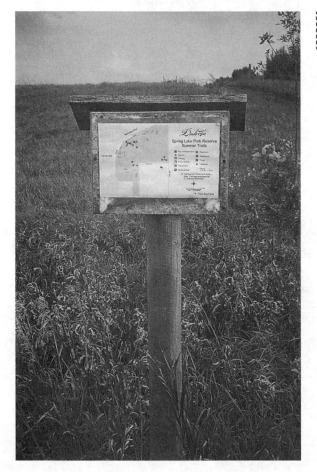

A typical trail sign at Spring Lake Park Reserve

0.29-mile bluff trail described above. You can continue straight ahead, but if you want to follow along the bluff, turn right, walk another few yards, and then turn left to follow the bluff trail. This is a short 0.17-mile loop—one of the best in the park!

If there is ever a trail museum, this stretch should be included as an example of the small deer-and-game trails from antiquity that original settlers would have used to traverse this undeveloped land. Its narrow, earthen, bare footpath is worn into the forest floor. It is also typical of the lacework of trails one expects to find woven through a birch-and-maple stand on the north shore. Occasionally a root snakes its way across your path and an exposed rock seems strategically placed smack-dab in the middle of the pathway.

It's quite a bit more rustic, less groomed, and not as fancy as the other trails in the park—and it's far, far too short! I was enjoying the trail so much that I had gone down half of it before I realized I had missed all the vistas overlooking the river and beyond. Several openings from the side of the trail give hikers splendid views of the river below and the outstretched valley to the northwest.

Rejoin the main trail from the bluff line, turn right, and continue back another 0.2 mile to the east end of the picnic shelter area.

There are wonderful, breathtaking vistas all along the edge of the park at this point. A carpet of lawn, seemingly held in place by stately oak trees, extends the entire length of this developed area. There is no trail, but if you continue along the edge of the bluff you eventually come to the lower half of the trail segment that loops out and back, first through more woodlands and then through patches of prairie at the western edge of the park.

About 0.16 mile south of the picnic shelter, there is a steep ravine cut from springs deep within the bluff itself. You have two trails from which to choose. The trail to the right cuts down into part of the ravine and back up the other side for a 0.3-mile segment. The left trail takes the high ground and pulls out into the edge of the meadowland to the east. Both of these two sections are less developed, and again a hiker can easily imagine and appreciate how trails have been developed over the centuries—from deer paths to mowed boulevards between the trees.

The two paths join, and once again you will parallel the river before coming out onto patchwork sections of prairie between small islands and corridors of trees, including a small stand of fine-needled white pines. Beyond is a farmstead—creating yet another image of bygone eras in this region.

The southern half of this loop drops down across the open, rolling hills of grassland before swinging up toward the developed area of the park. The first leg is 0.4 mile long. It meets up with an optional 0.74-mile loop that descends into the extreme southern portion of the park—away from the river.

Otherwise, the walking is casual from here on back. The trail continues on the loop that brought you along the park's southern portion.

This segment follows the gently rolling hills covered in meadow grasses that dominate the southern portions of the park. It winds along for 0.64 mile and reenters the picnic area by the parking lot.

NEARBY ACTIVITIES

Adjacent to this eastern section of the park is a separate airfield for remote-controlled model airplanes. The western unit of Spring Lake Park Reserve has a double-circle, walk-through archery range. The entrance to each area is on the main road, left (east) to the model-airplane field, or right (west) to the outdoor archery range.

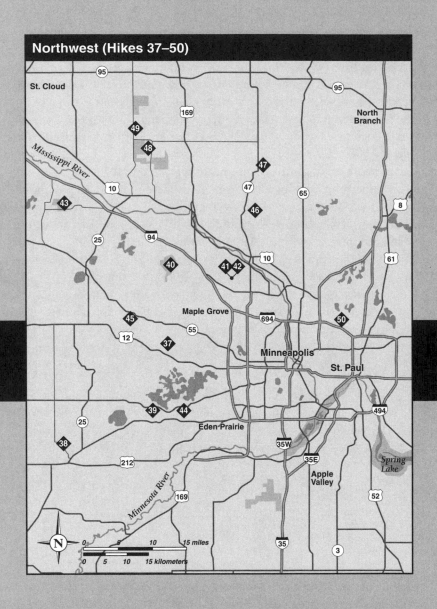

St. Cloud

95

169

95

North
Branch

Mississippi River

49

48

47

47

65

8

10

46

43

25

94

10

61

40

41 42

45

Maple Grove

55

694

50

12

37

Minneapolis

St. Paul

39 44

494

25

Eden Prairie

38

35W

35E

Spring
Lake

212

Apple
Valley

Minnesota River

169

52

35

3

N

0   5   10   15 miles

0   5   10   15 kilometers

NORTHWEST

37 BAKER PARK RESERVE

KEY AT-A-GLANCE INFORMATION

LENGTH: 6.2 miles

CONFIGURATION: Full circle

DIFFICULTY: Flat and easy with a few gradual inclines

SCENERY: A variety of forested areas, meadows, and only a brief glimpse of the lake

EXPOSURE: Mostly full sun; some shade

TRAFFIC: Popular trail for cyclists and runners, especially on weekends

TRAIL SURFACE: Paved

HIKING TIME: 2–2.5 hours

SEASON: Year-round (some trail segments convert to cross-country skiing in winter)

ACCESS: No fees

MAPS: Available at park headquarters or at threeriversparks.org

FACILITIES: Campground, picnic area, restrooms, pit toilets, boat rental, drinking water

SPECIAL COMMENTS: The shared hiking/biking trail has faster bike traffic at times, so be careful walking around corners and coming over rises in the trail.

CONTACT: (763) 694-7860

GPS TRAILHEAD COORDINATES

Latitude   N93° 38.285'

Longitude   W45° 1.250'

IN BRIEF

Woody highlands and evolving meadows and prairies are sprinkled throughout an otherwise marshy area around Lake Katrina. This 2,700-acre park reserve offers everything from golf and developed playgrounds to pathways skirting undeveloped marshlands.

DESCRIPTION

Like other parks past the western edge of the Twin Cities metro area, Baker Park Reserve's 2,700 acres lie atop the Des Moines ground moraine—a remnant of the Wisconsin ice age—which covers this entire region. Its rolling topography, myriad ice-block lakes, and maple–basswood-dominant forests are characteristics common to this part of Minnesota. Yet, like all other parks, Baker offers up its own personality to the intrepid hiker along its paved hiking/biking trails.

The entrance to the park is across the street from the trailhead, so park your vehicle and head back out the entrance and across County Road 29. You will see a trail spur on the right side of the roadway immediately upon entering that side of the park. Follow this short paved spur down through a dense stand of trees to the T intersection. Take the trail to the right, which will lead you through the entire southern half of the park. The trail, like other bike/hike loops, parallels the park's horse trail, but that trail is seldom visible and never crosses the hiking path.

Directions

From west Minneapolis, take US 12 West past Long Lake to CR 29 (Baker Park Road). Turn right (north), and follow the road for about 1.4 miles to the park entrance on the left.

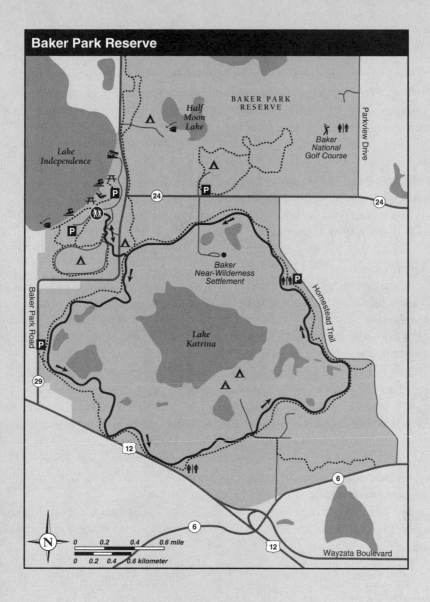

You immediately pass through a representative sampling of the trees you can expect to see throughout the park: basswoods, oaks, cottonwoods, and elms (only the maples are missing in this section). On your left will be the marshy areas that surround Lake Katrina in the distance. The trail snakes through stands of sumacs followed by open areas. Islands of trees are scattered along the modest hills upland from the lake.

At about 0.6 mile, the trail cuts sharply to the right and climbs around a small pond. From there it continues toward more marshy areas 0.25 mile farther. The trail finally straightens out a bit for the next 0.3 mile or so before reaching a trail spur to an alternate parking lot; here hikers and bikers can access the trail without going into the main part of the park.

I am not experienced enough to identify birds by their call, but I do recognize that different songs come from different birds—and the ever-present chorus of calls and chirps makes Baker Park Reserve a birder's challenge. For non-birders, the chorus proves delightful during the summer months.

As you continue, you'll notice that the vegetation along the trail constantly changes from marsh to field to forest. After the parking lot, you'll encounter aspens and more sumacs mixed in with what appear to be second- or third-generation growths of forest species.

The terrain becomes wetter at about the 1.5-mile mark, as indicated by islands of willows and more exposed vistas of the marshes and rush grass around the lake. All this will be on your left as you approach the boundary of the park and its proximity to US 12 just across the park's fenced border.

Shortly after leaving the fence behind, you'll get a good view of the lake. You will have hiked 2.5 miles at this point. The lake itself covers about 200 acres, while the boggy area surrounding it encompasses more than 225 acres of marshland. Three-tenths of a mile farther, there is a picnic area and a restroom, all underneath a power line that crosses overhead.

The Katrina Camp entrance road soon comes up on the right at about 3 miles. This road has recently been made part of the access route that now joins Baker Park Reserve with the popular Luce Line biking and hiking corridor, which runs extensively across the western reaches of the metro area.

The trail continues to wind around the southeastern edge of the lake, rising slowly from the marsh. You'll reach a rock bench at about 3.3 miles—a good resting point about halfway along the trail. About 0.25 mile farther, the trail drops down and passes a residential area bordering the park.

You'll come across a roadway leading left to the Trumpeter Swan Refuge. A resident flock of swans summers here, and around the third week of June the park hosts an interpretive program featuring these local trumpeters.

For the next mile or so, check out all the maples—some of the stands are impressive with towering, dominant trees reminiscent of the Big Woods growth seen in other regions around the Twin Cities. Just past this stand of maples, the trail intersects with a path leading to the administration offices across CR 24. If you want to add 1.5 miles to the hike, you can access the short hiking-only figure eight that begins at a spur by the administrative offices.

Staying on the main trail for another 0.3 mile will bring you past a shallow hillside with what appears to be an old landscape planting of both the indigenous and introduced plants that are currently scattered throughout the park. After another few tenths of a mile, the trail intersects the Baker Near-Wilderness Settlement. At this experiential learning site for school-age children, special-interest groups, and adult audiences, eight cabins serve as a residential living environment for program participants.

The road that intersects the trail crosses the highway and extends to the Marshview Group Camp. It crosses the designated hiking trail that forms a figure eight around the group camp and the area behind the administration building.

A bit farther, the trail passes through a stand of box elders on the right. This is also a rest stop for hikers and horses. At this point you are about 6 miles along the trail. Watch the side of the trail closely for the sign for the Oak Knoll Group Camp. Just a few yards past the group camp turn, you'll come upon the unmarked spur on the right that takes you out of the thicker woods and back to the entrance.

NEARBY ACTIVITIES

Check with the park office for activities at the Near-Wilderness Settlement or to get details on the hiking trail network behind the administrative office across CR 24. With access now open to the Luce Line trail corridor, determined trekkers can add another 30 miles to their agenda.

38 BAYLOR REGIONAL PARK

KEY AT-A-GLANCE INFORMATION

LENGTH: 4.6 miles

CONFIGURATION: Three loops off a main trailhead road

DIFFICULTY: Gently rolling and winding trails with gradual and modest rises in sections

SCENERY: Young maple forest with some larger trees; expansive marsh adjacent to shallow prairie lake

EXPOSURE: Cool shade under maples; exposed trails near lake

TRAFFIC: Moderate RV-camper use in summer; expect locals on weekends at picnic area and lake

TRAIL SURFACE: Some packed gravel in campground area; compacted earth otherwise

HIKING TIME: 1.25–2 hours at a casual pace

SEASON: Year-round

ACCESS: $5 daily vehicle fee; $24 annual vehicle fee

MAPS: At the barn headquarters

FACILITIES: Outhouse at trailhead near campground; other facilities at visitor center and within campground

SPECIAL COMMENTS: Hikers are likely to see a variety of migrating waterfowl in spring and summer at the marsh and in the lake areas.

CONTACT: (952) 466-5250 or tinyurl .com/baylorpark

GPS TRAILHEAD COORDINATES

Latitude   N93° 56.701'

Longitude   W44° 48.614'

IN BRIEF

This is a quaint, countylike park with a refreshing maple forest, marsh area, and modestly developed lakefront area. Whether you come to camp and hike or just spend a pleasant afternoon, Baylor offers a peaceful setting.

DESCRIPTION

The first impression one gets from entering Baylor Regional Park is that it's not really a park at all but a restored farm site. The large barn right across the parking lot that serves as the park's headquarters and the adjacent caretaker's residence seem reminiscent of a typical Midwestern homestead farm in Carver County.

The trail system meanders through nearly all of the park's 230 acres, providing hikers with great views of the lake, walks through thick maple stands, and a floating walkway across a marsh.

From the parking lot alongside the barn, walk between the two main buildings and head toward the campground. Utility camping will be on your left, but keep going to the first gravel road intersection. This is the start of Maple Trail. Take a left here, and walk past the second campsite—it's on your right—and head into the woods just past the bathhouse.

You will quickly see why it's called the Maple Trail. While not big, the maples are

----

Directions _____

Head west from Minneapolis on Crosstown 62 or I-494 to the intersection with US 212. Take US 212 west to MN 5. Take MN 5 west about 25 miles to Norwood, Minnesota. In Norwood, take CR 33 north 2.5 miles to park entrance on the right.

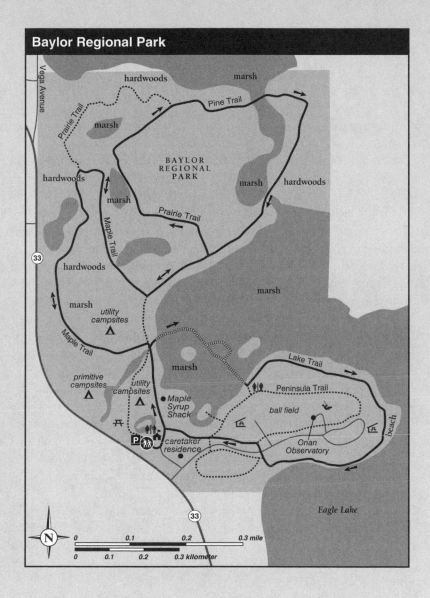

certainly plentiful. These are sugar maples; you can tell by the rounded inner corner of the lobes on the leaf (on red maples this corner forms a right angle). The trail runs fairly close to the highway as it heads north. At about 0.2 mile, it swings slightly west toward the highway but cuts back into more hardwoods, where older maples dominate. The path passes through a corridor of arched maple canopies to form a cool, shaded pathway.

At about 0.5 mile down the Maple Trail, you will come to an intersection on your right. This is the continuation of the Maple Trail back to the camping area. It is also a way to link up with the other major loop in this part of the park, so hang a right and enjoy more beautiful young and mature trees as the trail dips and curves through more sugar maples.

At the end of the Maple Trail, you will come out facing the marsh. You are now at the northern end of the campground road. Look for the Pine Trail on your immediate left, and take it. You will return on this section of the Pine Trail later. For now, follow the path as it skirts the marsh on your right for about 0.2 mile before you reach another fork. Take the left fork.

The trail at this point is called the Prairie Trail, and it cuts back into the woods. There are more wet areas in this section since elevations are lower. You will see a small pond, as well as a dense stand of mature maples in this section.

You will have traveled about 0.4 mile when the trail forms a T with the Pine Trail. Turn left, and you will return to the Maple Trail, but you want to turn right through more hardwoods (maples) and red pines as the trail meanders across the northernmost section of the park. There are some open, grassy areas on the right, and the larger marsh at the north end of Eagle Lake is on the left as the trail loops back to where it connects with the Prairie Trail again.

By this point you have taken two loops that have trailed through the wooded area of the park's western and northern reaches. As you meet up with the main trail, you will return to the end of the campground road where the trail forked earlier. If you backtrack past the campground on your right, you will come to a short spur on the left, right across the road from the second Maple Trail intersection. This spur leads to the Boardwalk Trail that crosses the marsh north of Eagle Lake.

The walkway is a floating trail that cuts across the western third of the marsh, putting the hiker a few feet above the water for a short 0.2-mile stretch. You can also walk the shoreline along the cattails and rushes for a good opportunity to enjoy the marsh from a close (but dry) vantage point.

The end of the boardwalk intersects with the Peninsula Trail to the right and the Lake Trail to the left. The Peninsula Trail loops through a developed recreational area of the park (with a playground, ball diamond, and more), while the Lake Trail follows the shoreline of Eagle Lake for about 0.9 mile. Opt for the Lake Trail.

For the first 0.25 mile, the marsh dominates the left side of the trail. Once you come upon the open water of Eagle Lake you'll be able to look out over this body of water for the next 0.4 mile or so. The trail will cut away from the lake and cross the road near the volleyball nets as it heads back toward the park's headquarters. It meets up with the main campground road right behind the caretaker's house across from the headquarters barn.

NEARBY ACTIVITIES

There's a lot to do at this quaint park. After hiking, you can enjoy a picnic or play a game of tennis or volleyball.

CARVER PARK RESERVE/LOWRY NATURE CENTER, Tamarack Trail

39

IN BRIEF

This trail meanders through all the represented ecosystems of the park—from oak forests to a watery network of lakes and marshes. The many interconnecting loop trails, all feeding from the Lowry Nature Center, provide for many short but resource-rich hikes.

DESCRIPTION

Carver Park Reserve covers more than 3,000 acres, one-third of which are interconnecting lakes, marshes, and sloughs. Yet one of the most diverse parts of Carver is represented in the area around the Lowry Nature Center, located in the heart of the park. This nature center has the distinction of being the first public environmental education center of its kind in the state. Its trail system offers a prime example of mixed woodland/marshland environment.

The park has an extensive trail system in its western section via horse-and-hiking trails that wind around three of the park's dozen large lakes. In addition, the eastern section offers more than 7.4 miles of bike/hike trails that wind between a half dozen more lakes. However, 5 or so miles of the interpretive trail system radiating out from the Lowry Nature Center in irregular loops are exclusively for hiking. While each segment is relatively short, these trails make up for it in their natural features and amenities.

KEY AT-A-GLANCE INFORMATION

LENGTH: 1.5-mile interpretive loop connected to optional segments

CONFIGURATION: Loop

DIFFICULTY: Very easy; mostly flat with several sections along boardwalks in the marsh areas

SCENERY: Lots of vistas of open water and marsh

EXPOSURE: Mostly sunny; some shade at beginning and end of hike

TRAFFIC: If the nature center is busy, expect the trails to be, too; otherwise there are enough trail spurs to find peace and quiet.

TRAIL SURFACE: Mostly wide, grassy trails; wooden walkways through marsh areas and Tamarack Trail loop

HIKING TIME: 1–1.5 hours

SEASON: Year-round

ACCESS: No fees

MAPS: Available at nature center or at threeriversparks.org (go to Carver Park Reserve, and click on "Lowry Nature Center" for a map specific to this trail)

FACILITIES: Nature center with restrooms, drinking water

SPECIAL COMMENTS: There is a great deal of natural history to learn about in a small area; the entire network can be explored in a day.

CONTACT: (763) 694-7650

GPS TRAILHEAD COORDINATES

Latitude   N93° 41.058'
Longitude   W44° 52.952'

Directions

Drive west on I-494 to MN 5 (Exit 11B); then go west about 10 miles to CR 11. Turn right (north) 2 miles to entrance to Lowry Nature Center. Go to end of nature center and park.

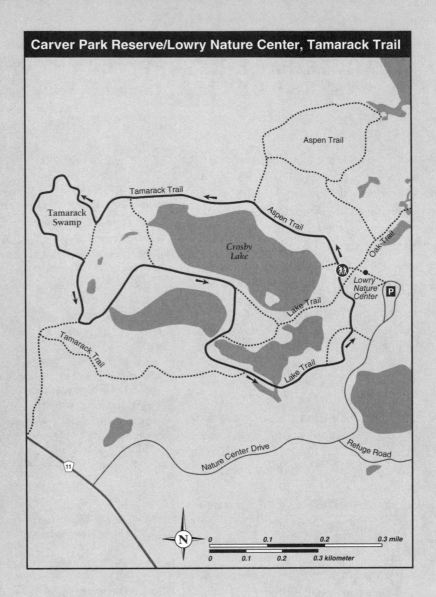

Carver Park Reserve/Lowry Nature Center, Tamarack Trail

Aspen Trail

Tamarack Trail

Tamarack
Swamp

Aspen Trail

Oak Trail

Crosby
Lake

Lowry
Nature
Center

P

Tamarack Trail

Lake Trail

Lake Trail

Nature Center Drive

Refuge Road

11

N

| 0 | 0.1 | 0.2 | 0.3 mile |

| 0 | 0.1 | 0.2 | 0.3 kilometer |

Beginning at the nature center (after you've spent time absorbing all the educational and informational displays and materials inside), take the Oak Trail toward the eastern end of Crosby Lake. This area is predominantly oak with stands of maples and basswoods. About 400 feet from the trailhead, the trail splits: Oak Trail veers to the right, and the Aspen Trail continues along the marsh grass and cattail shoreline of Crosby Lake. Take Aspen Trail at this point.

About 300 yards along the north shore of the lake, where the shoreline is especially marshlike, the Aspen Trail cuts out away from the lake to the right and continues on its own loop and interconnections. The trail along the lake beyond the intersection with the Aspen Trail is the beginning of the Tamarack Trail. Continue straight ahead and stay next to the lake. Go another 400 yards to another trail intersection that runs off to the left between Crosby Lake and a long, slender lake. That trail cuts back in a bit farther, but don't take it—there's a better route another couple of hundred yards ahead.

Just as you are exiting the woods, a trail to the right marks the origin of the 800-foot Tamarack loop. I found the tamaracks to be one of the most impressive features of this park. Tamaracks are quite common in northern Minnesota, but less so around the Twin Cities. They look like other evergreens in the summer with their spire-shaped growth and green needles. They lose their needles each fall just like the deciduous trees (oaks, maples, basswoods, ashes, and so on) lose their leaves. A tamarack can appear to be a dead spruce tree to the unknowing eye.

The trail drops down into a dense marshy area and becomes a 6-foot-wide boardwalk that snakes through islands of tamarack. Cattails and marsh grass are at your fingertips with no need for you to get wet—that's what attracted me to this area. There are few marshes with such diversity and accessibility. Usually you have to wait until winter when marshes freeze over to get this close. Here you can stroll along a wooden walkway right through the middle of this natural area at any time of the year with ease.

Here, in this tangled jumble of deadfall and swamp brush, everything appears to have fallen just as nature dictated. This is a very easy marsh to get to know, because you can walk through it and observe up close instead of standing on its periphery and looking in. I've always thought tamarack stands had a prehistoric look about them.

Bring your binoculars and keep an eye out through the tamaracks and grasses for redwing blackbirds and swamp sparrows, two of the more common birds in Minnesota's swamplands.

As you rejoin the Tamarack Trail on the western side of the lake, continue to the right. You'll spot a picnic table on a small knoll facing the lake and the country to the east. The trail continues along the high ground between Crosby Lake and the tamarack area before coming to a major intersection.

By mid-October, the park is beginning to get ready for winter and snowmobiling. The hiking trail is dwarfed by a 30-foot-wide, grass-mowed trail—a snowmobile highway, which cuts through the park and out onto the meadowlands to the left. This would be a good trail extension to take when wildflowers are in bloom.

Instead of staying on the Tamarack Trail, I opted to follow this grassy superhighway mainly because it led back between more lakes as it cut its swath through the grassy area south of Crosby Lake. This trail connects back up with Tamarack after dropping south of the lake areas about 0.5 mile farther along.

The north side of the trail provides open vistas across Crosby Lake and the oaks beyond. The terrain in the Carver Park area is a result of deposits of glacial till from the last ice age. The hills and rolling topography are examples of the ground moraine created by that ice age. These land formations and the vegetation covering them are considered some of the best examples of an undeveloped complex of wetlands/woodlands/old fields in the Hennepin County parks system.

Archaeological evidence indicates that the lands in and around the park were used as hunting and fishing grounds—but not for village or dwelling sites.

The park supports a diverse population of wildlife: deer, Canada geese, swans, beavers, minks, gray and red foxes, river otters, and a healthy population of songbirds. Minnesota's seemingly ubiquitous red-tailed hawk is a common inhabitant of the park as well. These lakes and adjoining meadows and woodlands create the perfect setting for attracting these and other critters.

Halfway around the south end of Crosby Lake, the trail dips south and cuts into the woods surrounding the smaller lake. A small wooden footbridge crosses a narrow section of the lake, adding a rustic touch to the trail.

This is Lake Trail, the southernmost trail in this section that forms a connecting loop going out and back from the center. Here the oaks are a little more mature, and there are a few more pockets of marshes. Just beyond the footbridge, an interpretive sign shares a bit of history about this particular area of the park.

In 1806, railroad tycoon James J. Hill, owner of the Great Northern Railroad, built a cutaway between Hopkins and Hutchinson—right through what is now this trail south of Crosby Lake. The tracks were removed in 1901, leaving this flat, straight section as the only reminder of events past.

After this historic area, the trail turns east and continues back through more trees bordering on a rolling meadow. Distant highway buzzing lets you know that you are still in an urban setting—but comfortably nestled in the environment of an active nature center. Another 300 yards, and the trail crosses another modest footbridge. Although the trail winds in and out of the woods, it remains flat and easy walking. Look for woodpeckers and chickadees in this section of the park. The trail continues on for about 400 yards to the hub of the trails at the Lowry Nature Center.

NEARBY ACTIVITIES

The Grimm Farm/Parley Lake area features both historic and natural amenities. The Wendelin Grimm Farm was a 137-acre tract that dates back to 1859. Grimm immigrated to Minnesota that year and spent the next few years developing a winter-hardy strain of alfalfa—the first ever developed in the United States. It was a significant leap toward the development of the dairy industry in the upper Midwest.

CROW-HASSAN PARK RESERVE 40

IN BRIEF

One of the biggest prairie-restoration projects in the park system, Crow-Hassan features expansive prairies above the slow-moving Crow River. Trails crisscross the meadows and then follow the river for much of its course adjacent to the park.

DESCRIPTION

Crow-Hassan Park offers a full range of natural amenities, from expansive, rolling prairie-like grasslands above the river valley to pockets of oaks and other hardwoods scattered along trails that wind out and back along the Crow River and ultimately return to the parking lot. When I hiked this park, the park map was apparently not up-to-date, since trails designated as hiking-only were also being used as horse trails. Whether this is new policy or not, I'm unsure, but each trail intersection is well marked with a hiker or horse icon labeling the appropriate use.

Hiking the designated horse trails presents a challenge: the trails are soft and ground into a fine, almost siltlike texture from all the hooves. This can make walking as tedious as tromping through loose sand. Still, there's opportunity to select several routes as you leave the prairie uplands and

KEY AT-A-GLANCE INFORMATION

LENGTH: 4.6 miles

CONFIGURATION: An irregular loop

DIFFICULTY: Easy; mostly flat or gently rolling, with a few steep but short inclines

SCENERY: Large expanses of prairie bordered by trees and dotted with lakes

EXPOSURE: Some shade in southern part of the park and along the river; full sun on the prairie

TRAFFIC: Peaceful along prairie trails and river; horse trails can be noisy

TRAIL SURFACE: Wide, earthen trail, some mowed lanes of grass

HIKING TIME: 1.5–2 hours

SEASON: Year-round; some designated ski-only trails in late fall and winter

ACCESS: No fees

MAPS: Available at park headquarters or at threeriversparks.org

FACILITIES: Primitive, with pit toilets and walk-in camping; no water

SPECIAL COMMENTS: This is a good park for a casual stroll. Don't be in a hurry; a stop along the river is a must.

CONTACT: (763) 694-7860

Directions

From the Twin Cities, take I-94 north to Rogers; take Exit 207 into town, and follow Main Street (CR 150) south 2 miles to CR 116, then north 2 miles to Hassan Parkway, west 2 miles to Park Road/Sylvan Lake Road (CR 203), and north to park entrance on left. Drive to first parking lot on right at the horse trailer staging area.

GPS TRAILHEAD COORDINATES

Latitude   N93° 37.794'
Longitude   W45° 11.097'

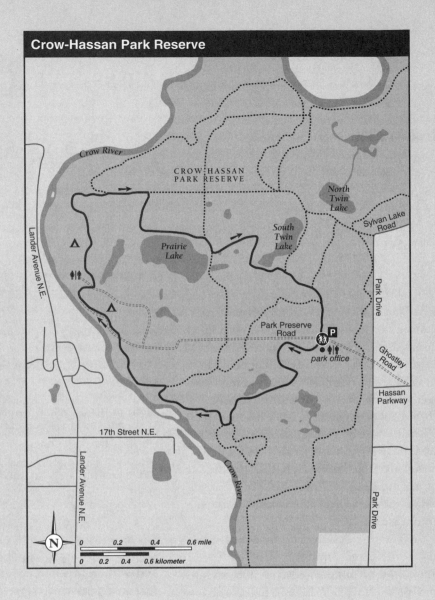

Crow River

CROW-HASSAN
PARK RESERVE

North
Twin
Lake

Sylvan Lake
Road

South
Twin
Lake

Prairie
Lake

Lander Avenue N.E.

Park Drive

Park Preserve
Road

P

park office

Ghostley
Road

Hassan
Parkway

17th Street N.E.

Lander Avenue N.E.

Crow River

Park Drive

N

| 0 | 0.2 | 0.4 | 0.6 mile |
| 0 | 0.2 | 0.4 | 0.6 kilometer |

make your way along the tranquil Crow River, which forms the western boundary of the park.

Leaving the parking lot just inside the main entrance (also the horse trailer staging area), follow the trail marked "hikers only" that leads south to the river. Keep on this main trail as it continues to drop to the edge of the river. Along the way, several trails appear on the left; ignore them. Once by the river, the trail turns into a horse trail and follows the river along its northwest/northern bank for about 0.4 mile. About 0.2 mile from where the trail first meets the river, a visible side path down a cut in the embankment leads to the river's edge and a gravel bar (at low water, at least) that stretches for several yards downstream. This is a great place to stop and view the river, have a picnic, and watch for canoeists paddling by. The Crow River is considered one of the foremost features of the park. Horse and hiking/pet trails follow most of its 7-mile western boundary. Farther downstream is a designated canoe takeout area for access to the park from the river.

Like most parks, Crow-Hassan serves as both a seasonal home and resting spot for scores of bird species on their migration to and from the northern regions. In the fall, the trees along the river are alive with blackbirds—hundreds and hundreds of them. Swans stop over in one of the lakes in the interior of the park.

After paralleling the riverbank for about 0.5 mile, the trail turns sharply for a short but steep uphill climb (about a 20-foot rise in elevation) where you will catch your first glimpse of the expansive prairie for which Crow-Hassan Park is renowned. This central prairie and a section farther north are part of a 480-acre prairie-restoration management area.

The trail levels off as it skirts the prairie and continues along the trees lining the top of the riverbank. A major hiking trail intersects here, and if you've bitten off more than you can chew, you can take this trail through the prairie and back to the parking area.

But most folks will elect to keep going along the river, which is bordered by a thick, continuous band of oaks. The surface of this trail turns to pea gravel (the trail is used by horses, too) as it continues along the upper slopes above the river. Ahead is a group camp in the guise of an old farm setting. The trail circles around this bit of development and once again joins the river. Here the trail passes through another corridor of oaks.

You can revel in the lushness of summer along these trails through dense corridors of maples and oaks. In comparison, late fall and winter hikers can enjoy an open understory and canopy, once leaves are shed, for long looks through the trees. Some trails look completely different from season to season.

As you circle around to the far western perimeter of the park, some of the trails become more like service roads—wide, grassy, rutted. There are two options for cutting back to the east. One is to stay to the left and follow the outside trail as it loops back at the northwest corner. Another option is to take the roadlike lane to the right, which is one of the old Red River oxcart routes used prior to railroads in the area. This is the only section of the oxcart trail that ties into this particular hike, so I decided to take it for 0.25 mile to the east, where I connected with the hiking trail again.

This trail leads trekkers right through the heart of an upland prairie with a mantle of flowing grasses and the occasional renegade tree. An Adirondack-like shelter sits above Prairie Lake, where you'll find a table and a stove for four-season use. The trail follows the north shore of Prairie Lake. The area immediately to the north and northeast is the most complete example of the prairie plant community. In 1968, naturalists discovered an ungrazed and untilled borrow pit, which showed a profile of the undisturbed prairie prior to agricultural use by the early settlers. This led to Three Rivers' prairie restoration and management efforts in the park.

In the fall, keep your eyes open for large, white birds on the far shore of the lake. You may very well see a few trumpeter swans resting on their journey south along the Mississippi flyway corridor. Other birds to watch for are meadowlarks, grasshopper sparrows, vesper sparrows, pileated woodpeckers (they leave a rectangular hole in dead trees), and red-tailed hawks, probably the most common hawk in Minnesota.

The trail continues along the northern end of the lake and up to an intersection with a service road. Take a right on the service road, and hike for about 200 yards to where the hiking trail intersects on the left. Take that left to remain on the hiking loop. For the next 0.7 mile, the trail meanders over and through even more prairie as it skirts past islands of aspen, maple, and birch. At about 0.3 mile along this section, South Twin Lake can be seen to the north.

The trail climbs and winds its way back through a small island of trees before gradually ascending through a wooded area behind the parking lot and horse staging area.

NEARBY ACTIVITIES

Lake Rebecca Park Reserve, where paddle and hiking opportunities abound, is only 8.3 miles upstream from Crow-Hassan Park.

ELM CREEK PARK RESERVE

IN BRIEF

King of the trails in this book for sheer mile-age covered, the Elm Creek trail offers a grand route through mostly unspoiled Minnesota countryside. There are marshes, hardwood forests, lots of meadows, and plenty of room to stretch your hiking legs. If you've got the time and want to spend a good half day hiking, this is the trail for you.

DESCRIPTION

With more than 4,900 acres within the park's boundary, Elm Creek Park Reserve naturally represents one of the longest hiking loops in the state. The 10-mile Hayden-Lemans Lake loop encircles most of the northern half of the park. This same area is ground moraine of the Des Moines lobe of the Wisconsin ice age glacial material. The combined watershed of this area drains more than 70,000 acres, nearly one-third of Hennepin County. It is through this expansive drainage area that this paved hiking trail leads.

For parking convenience, start at the lot at the Eastman Nature Center and follow the road up to Elm Creek Road and the park's entrance. From there, go right a couple of hundred yards to the trailhead of Elm Creek Trail.

Directions

From Minneapolis, head north on I-494. Continue west when it becomes I-94 again for about 3 miles to the exit ramp for 93rd Avenue North. Take 93rd Avenue North to the right (east) for about 1 mile to Fernbrook Lane (CR 121). Turn left, and go another mile to Elm Creek Road. Turn right into the park, and follow the road to the park entrance on the right. Continue down toward the nature center and park.

KEY AT-A-GLANCE INFORMATION

LENGTH: 11.25 miles

CONFIGURATION: A fat, crescent-shaped loop with several side-spur options

DIFFICULTY: Mostly flat and even with a few long but moderate grades to conquer

SCENERY: A showcase of central Minnesota, from marshes to maples, fields to forests

EXPOSURE: Both shade and full sun; be prepared on hot days

TRAFFIC: Not too crowded once away from the nature center complex

TRAIL SURFACE: Paved throughout since it doubles as a bike route

HIKING TIME: 3.5–4.5 hours

SEASON: Year-round; some segments double as ski trails in winter.

ACCESS: No fees

MAPS: Available at park headquarters or at threeriversparks.org

FACILITIES: Restrooms and drinking water at the center; nothing along the hike—you are on your own.

SPECIAL COMMENTS: Bring snacks and water; few places are designated for rest stops, so pick your own along the way.

CONTACT: (763) 694-7894

GPS TRAILHEAD COORDINATES

Latitude   N93° 26.900'

Longitude   W45° 9.490'

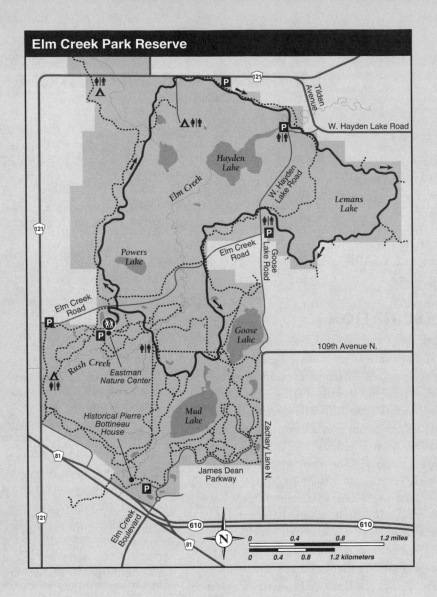

The trail is paved, 10 feet wide, and well maintained throughout the hike. It starts out along a shallow hogback ridge bordered by grasslands. The trail meanders through the wooded, hilly area. A stand of maples with a sumac understory will be on your right before you cut through a marsh area with many willows, dogwoods, and, of course, marsh grasses and cattails. These are but a few of the many wetland basins in this part of the park. You'll see representative cattail marshes, sedge meadows, and tamarack swamps, all bordered by woodlands or grassy meadows typical of the more open prairie.

At about 1.5 miles, you'll cross a wooden footbridge as the trail continues through marshy areas. There are some big woods nearby. In fact, a sanctuary of Big Woods forest is preserved in the northwest section of the park—and not accessible to visitors. Many wild turkey sightings are reported here. Several trail spurs—mostly snowshoe trails used during the winter—also veer off the main trail.

After the footbridge, the horse trail that has been running parallel to the left of the hiking trail crosses over and parallels on the right side as the features of the park turn into more open areas with more wetlands. The trail is on a gradual incline at this point. For the next 0.25 mile it will wind its way through alders and dogwoods on the right, and more wooded areas on the left. You are basically skirting the wetlands around Hayden Lake to the east and an unnamed lake nearer you, also to the east.

At the extreme northern end of the main park, the trail runs smack into County Road 121 and parallels this road for nearly 0.25 mile. There are several parking areas on CR 121 for those who wish to hike only these northern segments.

At the Hayden Lake Group Camp road, hikers are about a third of the way along this loop. The trail follows a power line for this section, through open country with scattered stands of aspens, some eastern cedars, and open expanses of grasslands.

You will be reminded at the trailhead that there are no facilities along the entire 10-mile stretch. I saw no toilets, no drinking water, and only one picnic table. You will find several places to stop along the way for a light picnic, however. At high noon in summer this trail could become very hot. It's a 10-foot-wide black bituminous surface with shade available only in islands of trees off the trail.

After paralleling the highway, the trail turns abruptly south and crosses a footbridge at Hayden Creek. If you want, venture up the creek toward Hayden Lake to possibly see a flower for which the area is well known—Minnesota's state flower, the showy lady's slipper.

You have several options to shorten your hike at this point. You can take the Lake Road to the right and cut nearly 2 miles off this hike or opt for the horse trail to eliminate about 1.5 miles. Both of these options pass through an area listed as having Indian burial mounds. Whether these mounds are particularly discernible or not is something you'll have to discover on your own.

Staying on the main trail past this juncture, you'll cross under the power line again. The trail takes a steep uphill climb just past the power lines at Hayden Lake and then continues along the upland prairie area of the park. Here the path skirts the extreme eastern boundary of the park, and the residential and commercial area of the town of Champlain comes into view. A handful of trail spurs lead into Champlain, where you can access several convenience stores to get some refreshments. There is also a lone picnic table sitting on a knoll at one of these spurs.

Back on the trail, continue past an unnamed lake on the left (Lemans is on the right), through larger trees in a more mature wooded area with more open spaces. There are more houses in this area, too, but at least now there are mature oaks and maples through which you can walk and not focus on someone's backyard.

The trail climbs out of the lowlands, past more houses and more trail spurs. It keeps ascending slowly but steadily as you go first south, then west. Shortly after the trail turns to the north, you will intersect Goose Lake Road and the horse trail. At this point you are about two-thirds of the way along this trail. Cross the road and follow the trail as it heads west, then slowly curves left to go south. You will intersect Elm Creek Road 0.7 mile after leaving the last road crossing. If you are starting to tire and want to shorten the hike, turn right along the horse trail or follow Elm Creek Road about 2 miles to the park's entrance. Otherwise, continue south across the road for the last 3-mile section of trail.

Turn right at the next intersection, and follow the signs back toward the Nature Center. This takes you along the western shore of Goose Lake. At the southern end of the lake is yet another intersection. The trail to the left runs between Goose and Mud lakes and meanders through the southern half of the park—that trail is another day's hike in its own right. Instead, head right, following the signs that direct you to Mud Lake. It's about 2.5 miles to the Nature Center.

The trail actually follows a hogback ridge above the northern end of Mud Lake before climbing up along yet another ridge that is lined with sumacs, making a nice corridor through which to hike. At the top of the ridge sits another lone picnic table with a nice view of the lake. When you first approach it, Mud Lake appears to be a marshy wetland only. Rising up to the ridge, you realize that the southern half of the lake actually contains water.

The trail continues along the lake until it intersects with a trail that directs hikers back toward the Nature Center—now only 1.2 miles away. Once on these trails, you will find many spurs that all eventually lead back to the center. Many of these are interpretive trails that the Eastman Nature Trail hike (see facing page) explores.

The main trail and the horse trail converge at the creek crossing. This is Elm Creek again, cutting its way across the park. From here, it's a steady uphill climb to the upper meadows just east of the park's entrance. You will come out almost across the road from the trailhead you took 10 miles earlier. From here, follow a gentle downhill loop to the main parking lot.

NEARBY ACTIVITIES

The Eastman Nature Center has such an extensive interpretive trail system that I've separated it as a hike unto itself. If you're up to it, there are several more miles of great trails to hike. Or try the route around Mud Lake.

ELM CREEK PARK RESERVE,
Eastman Nature Trail

42

IN BRIEF

A 13,000-square-foot nature center is being reconstructed at the Elm Creek Park Reserve. It is scheduled to reopen in the late summer of 2012.

Eastman Nature Trail lies at the heart of the Elm Creek Park Reserve, the largest park in the metro area. Each lobe of the trail system showcases the best this park offers.

DESCRIPTION

The Eastman Nature Trail hike is the shorter of two hikes in this book (see Elm Creek Park Reserve, page 179) that are located in the area's largest metro park. This interpretive trail is a good primer on the diversity of the area's ecosystem and definitely complements the other, longer hike, should you want to combine the two for a day's worth of hiking.

Begin your hike right out the back door of the nature center. Follow the signs to the Meadowlark Trail along a well-marked, wood-chip path. You will be walking through a dense stand of sugar maples, up a gradual incline to the Sumac-Meadowlark Trail junction. Take the left-hand trail toward Meadowlark.

A short distance beyond this junction, on your right, is a grass pathway known as

Directions

From Minneapolis, head north on I-494. Continue west for about 3 miles, where the interstate becomes I-94 again, to the exit ramp for 93rd Avenue North. Take 93rd Avenue North to the right (east) for about 1 mile to Fernbrook Lane (CR 121). Turn left, and go another mile to Elm Creek Road. Turn right into the Elm Creek Park Reserve, and follow the road to the park entrance on the right. Continue down toward the nature center and park.

KEY AT-A-GLANCE INFORMATION

LENGTH: 3.8 miles

CONFIGURATION: Irregular figure eight

DIFFICULTY: A few elevation changes, but basically level and easy

SCENERY: Meadows, hardwood forests, ponds, and creek beds

EXPOSURE: Sun and shade intermixed throughout; mostly shade in creek area

TRAFFIC: This is a very popular center, but a multitude of paths provide trails for everyone

TRAIL SURFACE: Mowed grass; earthen trail

HIKING TIME: 1.5–2 hours

SEASON: Probably best enjoyed early spring–late fall; could turn into a winter wonderland with snow

ACCESS: No fees

MAPS: Available at park headquarters or at threeriversparks.org (click on "Elm Creek Park Reserve")

FACILITIES: Restrooms and drinking water at the center

SPECIAL COMMENTS: If you're going to take the Elm Creek Trail or others in the more remote reaches of the park, bring snacks and water.

CONTACT: (763) 694-7894

GPS TRAILHEAD COORDINATES

Latitude   N93° 26.985'

Longitude   W45° 9.325'

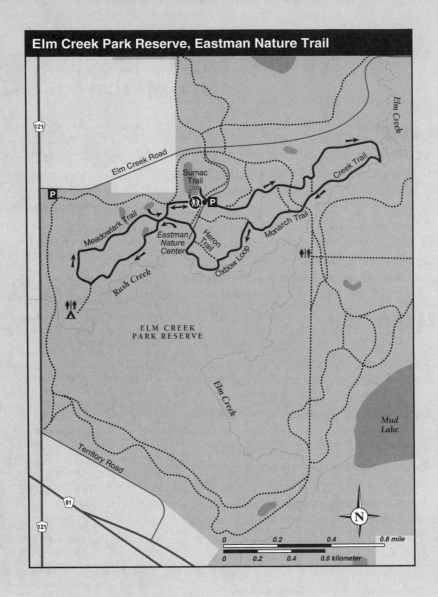

the Landscape for Wildlife trail. This short interpretive trail explains the practice of planting bushes and shrubs that attract birds and other wildlife. Some of the varieties along this trail and throughout the park include wild plum, hazelnut, and black chokecherry. You will take this trail later when you can use it to join up with the next connecting loop.

Another short distance beyond the Landscape spur, the trail forks again. Stay to the left and walk clockwise around this large meadow along Rush Creek.

The meadow is dotted with young aspen trees. It will also introduce you to a species that seems to be very prevalent in this park—the prickly ash! This is a nasty, small, treelike plant similar to a young ash sapling in size and appearance. However, the stems and branches have roselike thorns that can pierce your skin, rip your clothing, and give you a most miserable time of cutting through the understory. Prickly ash is common here and in other parks in this part of Minnesota.

The trail has become an earthen pathway through this old meadow that also contains box elders and ashes. It winds through a thicket of these species before arriving at a bench that provides a view over the meadow. A short distance from the bench, the trail swings down toward Rush Creek and follows it for about 0.25 mile. This low-lying area tends to flood in the spring, judging from the number of sand deposits and grass strands laced throughout the lower branches of the alders growing here.

At the top of the Meadowlark loop, you will come to a trail that leads to the Rush Creek Group Camp. From here the trail leads back into the woods as it rises up perhaps 30 to 40 feet out of the lower meadow-and-creek area along a trail that is again covered in wood chips.

Next, the trail turns into a grassy corridor through a thicketlike growth of sumacs, ashes, and box elders. The trail skirts the upland edge of the meadow as it climbs through a transition zone between the lowlands of the creek bed and the upper zone of maples and hardwoods. Basswood trees are more common now as the trail winds through islands of trees and across small meadowlike openings and grasslands.

You will come upon another bench, on the right, that looks down through a narrow corridor of bushes to the meadow below. The trail continues on, cutting through more prickly ash and sumac before opening up on another meadow on the left. If you are hiking in the late spring, about 150 yards beyond the bench on the left, look for the beautiful blooms of a wild crab apple tree right alongside the trail.

The trail passes through an area with marshes on both sides, some with open water. These ponds are great places to watch for migrating waterfowl and summer lake dwellers such as great blue herons and great white egrets.

As the trail veers to the right, you can get a better view of the pond on your right. A few hundred yards later, you return to the previously hiked feeder trail. Look for the intersection with the Landscape for Wildlife loop shortly thereafter on your left; take it.

The Landscape trail is only a few hundred yards long. It cuts sharply to the right and connects at a T intersection with the Sumac Trail. Take the Sumac Trail to the left, and follow the signs to the boardwalk. You will come upon another intersection with a bike trail marked "To Landscape Trail," but stay on the Sumac Trail and keep heading toward the boardwalk. Looking through the trees, you can see the lake and boardwalk ahead, so keep it in your sights.

As you approach the lake, check out this forest. You'll see basswoods, maples, and oaks. This stand is younger and thicker than other stands you've been through. It's also the site of branch-breaking, tree-tearing 125-mph winds that ripped through here in the early 1980s. As you look at the forest floor, you can still see some of the larger trunks of trees that were knocked over during that blast of wind.

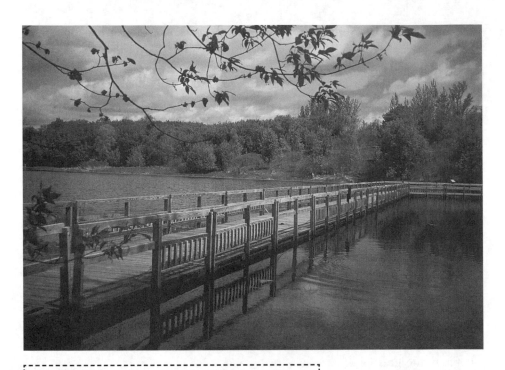

The Boardwalk Trail spans the pond at Eastman Nature Center.

The boardwalk trail spans the open pond. Step onto the boardwalk quietly, and you might see a painted turtle sunning itself on the logs and floating mats of debris on the left. It's also common to see summer visitors of Canada geese in ponds and lakes, so check out the far end of this pond while out on the boardwalk.

Upon leaving the boardwalk, take the trail to the right; then cross the main park entrance road. Just after crossing the paved roadway, there is a trail to the Outdoor Classroom on your left. This is the trail you want to take to continue along the outer interpretive loop of trails.

You will walk right past the classroom circle in a clearing just off the main road. Look for a grassy trail going up a hill at the other end of the open circle. This spur intersects with the Monarch Trail to the east. If the spur isn't readily visible, just stay on the current trail; it, too, connects with the Monarch Trail just a few yards farther down. In either case, once you intersect with the Monarch Trail, turn left.

As you wind up and around on the trail, you will pass under silver maples and box elders before coming out onto the open meadow. Cresting a knoll, you may see signs of a past controlled burn of these grasslands. The burns occurred in early spring 2001. The area on the left side of the walkway had been burned earlier, so you can compare the two sides to see how fast it takes for Mother Nature to regenerate after a prairie fire.

The path winds across these meadows as it flows up and down over gentle swells in the grassland. More burned areas appear on the left beyond a bench perched near the highest point on this vast prairielike area.

As you come down the far side of the meadow, the wide grassy trail forms a right-angle intersection (to your right) with a trail that heads back down to the creek. Keep going straight. A few yards farther, and you will cross the paved bike trail. If you wish to add the 11.3-mile loop hike through the rest of Elm Creek Park Reserve, turn left here and follow descriptions for Elm Creek (see page 179). Otherwise, cross the paved trail and stay on the main course for another 0.1 mile or so until you come to the T intersection with the Creek Trail. Take a left, and follow the trail up through the meadow for about 0.5 mile before dropping south to another T intersection. Take the trail to the right along Rush Creek.

You are now heading back to the visitor center. The Creek Trail rejoins the Monarch Trail (keep left). You'll be walking under some of the biggest, tallest maples in the park along this corridor. About 0.2 mile farther, you will reach another fork in the trail. Keep left again to enjoy the outer loop, called the Heron Trail. Another 0.2 mile, and it will fork again, this time joining the Oxbow Loop. Take the left again and explore the bottomlands of Rush Creek. You pass under huge cottonwoods and basswoods in this area.

At a sharp bend in the creek, you'll find a bench and short fence defining an observation area. Beyond this point are several wooden footbridges over the creek. This area can be buggy after spring floods. After several bridges, you'll see a series of big birdhouse-type structures. These are wood-duck nesting boxes.

The trail rises a bit, and the forest becomes maples and oaks again. The trail rejoins the Heron Trail for a short segment before it connects with the main trail about 50 yards from the trailhead behind the visitor center.

NEARBY ACTIVITIES

The entire park spans more than 4,900 acres, so the trail network is quite extensive. Options include many more miles of trails both north and south of the nature center complex of trails.

43 LAKE MARIA STATE PARK

KEY AT-A-GLANCE INFORMATION

LENGTH: 3.9 miles

CONFIGURATION: Serpentine loop

DIFFICULTY: Easy to moderate; hilly throughout, but rises and descents are gradual.

SCENERY: Very woodsy with many oaks; fabulous in fall

EXPOSURE: Some open areas; most sections under canopy; short section north of road could get hot in full sun

TRAFFIC: Heaviest on southern half except around Bjorkland Lake; eastern edge is less developed, with only trails.

TRAIL SURFACE: Earthen trails, easily marked; some gravel road surfaces

HIKING TIME: 1.5–2 hours

SEASON: Year-round; best in summer and fall

ACCESS: Minnesota State Park fee system: $5 daily, $25 annual permit, $12 annual permit for disabled individuals

MAPS: Available at park headquarters or at www.dnr.state.mn.us /state_parks/lake_maria

SPECIAL COMMENTS: This park is particularly popular with students from St. Cloud State University.

CONTACT: (763) 878-2325

GPS TRAILHEAD COORDINATES

Latitude   N93° 56.478'

Longitude   W45° 18.823'

IN BRIEF

The trails that weave through Lake Maria (pronounced Ma-RYE-ah) State Park take hikers through many samples of Minnesota's natural history: remnants of the Big Woods, marshes, and glacier-formed potholes. Noted for its wildlife, including an endangered species of turtle, and a stopping-off point for trumpeter swans, Lake Maria offers a full menu of sights as well as secluded backpacking on winding trails through oak forests.

DESCRIPTION

The trail starts at the western end of the visitor center. This path passes south through a rolling forest of oaks and maples. You immediately get the sense that Lake Maria is a special park. After 0.3 mile, when you come to a trail intersection, continue straight ahead.

As you progress, you will notice that the trail winds its way up and down small hills and knolls—remnants of ages past. These are deposits of the St. Croix glacial moraine formed during the Wisconsin ice age. About halfway down, a thick canopy of golden leaves still clings to the trees, even toward the end of fall. There is little understory along the first sections of this trail, which translates into clear

Directions

Take I-94 north to the *second* Monticello exit (Exit 193). Go right to West Sixth Street/Pine Street, then left about seven blocks to Elm. Take a right, and travel one block to CR 39. Follow CR 39 west back over I-94 and continue about 7 miles to CR 11; turn right (north) and go about 1.5 miles. Turn left into the park entrance, go past the information office, and then take your next left. Drive to the trail center at the end of the road.

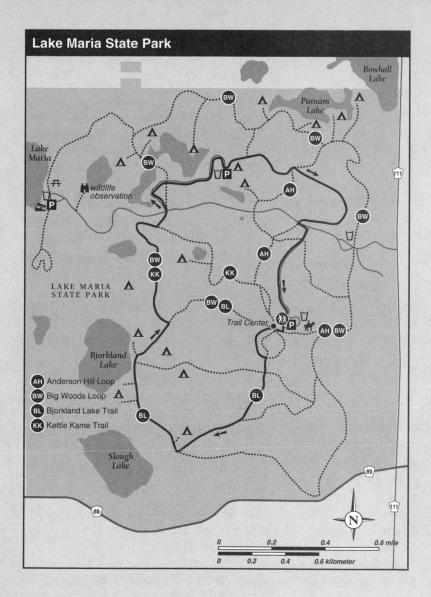

Lake Maria State Park

Bowhall Lake

Putnam Lake

Lake Maria

wildlife observation

LAKE MARIA STATE PARK

Bjorkland Lake

(AH) Anderson Hill Loop
(BW) Big Woods Loop
(BL) Bjorkland Lake Trail
(KK) Kettle Kame Trail

Trail Center

Slough Lake

| 0 | 0.2 | 0.4 | 0.6 mile |

| 0 | 0.2 | 0.4 | 0.6 kilometer |

N

views of this oak forest and the gently rolling terrain. By late fall, the forest floor is a dense, but loose, carpet of oak leaves—a sea of parchmentlike leaf patterns you have to wade through along the trail. It can be fun walking with the rustling leaves, but be careful—they hide depressions, exposed roots, and the occasional toe-thumping rock, all buried beneath a mantle of golden browns.

As the trail ascends along the top of an oak-covered knoll, Campsite 17, the first of several remote backpacker campsites in the area, comes into view. Set back into the woods off the main trail, each campsite is a simple cleared area with a table and a spot to pitch a tent. Placed about 40 yards apart, campsites are screened by bushes and have numbered pathways that lead off the main trail.

At this point, the hiking trail ends and the horse trail begins. Where the trail Ts, take a right (past Campsite 16) and head north. The trail drops down off the knoll and cuts through a small stand of aspens on this 0.5-mile stretch to the lake. Campsites 14 and 15 are at the bottom of the knoll, just before the trail reaches an open meadow. Beyond the meadow lies Bjorkland Lake. A trailhead at the canoe access point on the lake offers hikers two alternatives: head back to the right through the woods to the visitor center, or continue on the horse trail for access to the northern part of the park.

Although I generally prefer not to hike on horse trails, I did decide to continue on this one north from Bjorkland Lake. It's a narrow corridor flanked by oaks. Shortly you will see a hiking trail going straight. Turn left to stay on the horse trail. Soon you will come upon Campsite 7, which sits on a hill overlooking a marshy region below. The trail climbs and dips along this section—more glacial moraine deposits. Elevation varies by about 20 feet in this area. The meandering path climbing up through the oaks really heightens the sense that you have indeed embarked on a hike through the woods. It's this rough, wooded terrain, altered by the terminal moraine topography, that truly adds character to Lake Maria.

Past Campsite 7 0.5 mile, you will intersect the park road that connects the entrance to the boat launch and picnic area on Lake Maria about 0.4 mile to the west. If your trek takes you to Lake Maria, set aside some time to enjoy the boardwalk leading to the Zumbrunnen Interpretive Trail. It measures about 0.75 mile long out and back and offers fascinating information on the natural and cultural resources of the area.

Cross this road and head to the entrance to the Primitive Camp Group parking area. Just follow the road past the marshy lake on your left. In these and other spots where the marsh is close to the road, be on the lookout for a special turtle—one with yellow dots on its back. This is one of the few parks in which you'll see this threatened species in Minnesota, called Blanding's turtle.

You'll come to a split in the trail. The left spur goes about 0.3 mile across the marsh to one of two rental camping cabins in the park ($27.50 per night; reservations needed). Continue to the edge of the parking lot, where the trail heads back into the woods. A short distance up the trail, another spur takes off to the left. It leads to another remote rental cabin, this one on the shore of Putnam Lake on the north boundary of the park, as well as more tent sites at the Putnam Lake backpacking area.

A little more than 0.3 mile from the last junction, a horse trail cuts through this route. For a side trip you can follow it to the left to find a network of loops and other trail segments, including a hike up to Anderson Hill's scenic overlook. Otherwise, stay on the main trail—the hiking-only trail—as it works its way along a ridgeline.

At what appears to be the highest point along this ridge trail, just as the trail swings back south toward the road, you'll find a bench. Aptly placed, it provides a limited panorama of the wooded ravine at the base of the ridge on the opposite side of the trail. This bench marks the site of a good example of the way that animals cope in the winter when there is a shortage of food. Look behind the bench at the stand of trees with the dark-gray, flaky bark. These are ironwood trees. If you have trouble identifying them, look about 2.5 feet up their trunks from the ground, and notice that the bark has been scraped off. Now, look more closely—those are teeth marks. If you check the trees in a 50-foot-radius circle, you will find similar markings. It is probable that the snow was this deep here, limiting access to vegetation on the forest floor. Thus, animals had to gnaw at the trees available above the snow line, eating the cambium layer beneath the bark. Perhaps deer find ironwood particularly tasty—or they were particularly hungry.

The trail continues around the top of the ravine and then gradually makes its way back to the main park road. You can cross at this point and follow the visitor center road back to the parking lot or continue along the horse trail through the woods. Once you cross the road, it's a 0.4-mile hike back to the parking lot and visitor center.

NEARBY ACTIVITIES

Lake Maria connects with Silver Lake for a short but relaxing opportunity to enjoy canoeing.

44 LAKE MINNEWASHTA REGIONAL PARK, Marsh Trail Loop

KEY AT-A-GLANCE INFORMATION

LENGTH: 1.3 miles, with options for shorter loops

CONFIGURATION: Balloon

DIFFICULTY: Mostly easy; a few steep hills require moderate effort, but other elevation changes are gradual.

SCENERY: A pleasant, shallow bay in a woodsy setting

EXPOSURE: Entire trail is shaded.

TRAFFIC: Primarily used by those in the immediate residential area

TRAIL SURFACE: Narrow; some mowed sections

HIKING TIME: 1–1.25 hours

SEASON: Year-round; summer trails perhaps a little more crowded

ACCESS: $5 daily permit, $24 annual; available through Carver County

MAPS: Usually available on-site; otherwise through Carver County Parks

FACILITIES: Developed area of park has restrooms, drinking water, picnic areas, and parking lot.

SPECIAL COMMENTS: It's like a sampler hiking area, with most of the amenities of bigger parks and more diverse terrain.

CONTACT: (952) 466-5250 or tinyurl .com/lakeminnewashta

GPS TRAILHEAD COORDINATES

Latitude   N93° 35.435'
Longitude   W44° 25.599'

IN BRIEF

The park is but a small corner of a not-so-big lake, yet for shorter hikes that offer moderate changes in elevation and pleasant scenery, it's a good choice for an enjoyable outing. Woods are characteristic oaks, maples, and other hardwoods. The outer-trail loop is trisected for myriad hiking course variables.

DESCRIPTION

Lake Minnewashta offers two trail systems. The larger system is in the western and southern halves of the park, also the place where all the development has occurred. The northern section of the park provides a more primitive setting for hiking.

The Marsh Trail, the object of this hike, is the longest of the three loop sections at Lake Minnewashta. Begin at the parking lot and follow the general shoreline of the lake. There's no sandy beach here, but there are plenty of the marshy grasses and cattails common to rural lakes and prairie ponds. If you look straight out across the bay, you will see that both entrances to this elongated bay are low, marshy areas.

For about the first 300 yards, the trail is a straight shot through oaks, ashes, and maples, as you would expect in this part of

----

Directions

From Chanhassen, drive west on CR 5 toward the Minnesota Arboretum. Go right (north) on Hazeltine Boulevard (CR 41) about 1.5 miles to park entrance on left. Upon entering park, turn left and follow the road for about 300 yards to the first picnic area/parking lot on the right. The trailhead is at the far end of the parking lot. Take the trail that follows the lake.

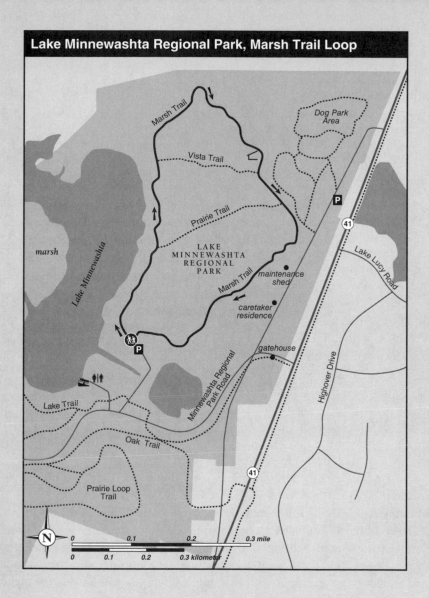

Minnesota. As the trail approaches a bay at the northeast end of the lake, look around at all the stately oaks. They are a bit gnarly, but that just adds character to their profile. As you look out over the lake at this point, you will be able to see some of the many houses built on the far shore beyond the bay.

The trail climbs about 40 feet above the lake to a ridgeline, where you will come to the intersection with the Prairie Trail. The Prairie Trail cuts inland from the lake for about 400 yards and meets up with the Marsh Trail again near the top of the ridge, making possible a shorter 0.8-mile loop. In the winter this route is popular with cross-country skiers. These trails are clearly marked at trailheads.

Continuing along the main perimeter trail, you are still following the general shoreline of the lake. The trail becomes a little more demanding as it follows the irregular topography. It also continues to ascend as it traces the ridge north. Maples, oaks, and even a few black cherry trees are the main species in these higher reaches on the slopes above the lake. Hiking becomes a bit more moderate as the trail continues to climb to about 80 feet above the lake.

Another 300 yards beyond the Prairie Trail junction is the turnoff to Vista Trail. This is the second opportunity to cut across to the other side of the Marsh Trail. It shortens the distance of the full outer loop by almost 0.5 mile.

At the top of the loop on the Marsh Trail, there are several smaller, earthen paths that lead off this main trail to the north. Here the trail winds its way through the upland woodlands as it continues to climb slightly along the way. It then starts to turn back down the other side of the loop and head south through more oaks and maples.

Soon you will come upon a shelter on the left. This appears at first to be the high point on the park trail, but that's still ahead. On rivers they call a false headland on the shore "point no point." This part of the trail could be called "top no top" because it soon becomes apparent that there is still a little more uphill hiking to do. However, a bench and drinking water here make this a good place to stop.

It's about another 400 yards to the junction with the upper Vista Trail. After this, you have less than 300 yards to the Prairie Trail junction on the right. A new dog-trail section featuring a mile of trails has been added just off the upper end of the loop. The highest point in the park (as best as I could determine from the faint topo lines on the map) is about 200 yards past the Prairie Trail. Here you come upon a small, but welcome, stand of white pines.

The trail appears to climb slightly beyond this point. There is a maintenance shed about 100 yards past what the map shows as the highest contour line (1,000 feet) in the park. Another 300 yards and the caretaker's home is off to the left.

The trail reaches an open meadow—one of those oak prairie areas. Ash trees are scattered throughout this section, while a small stand of cedar trees contrasts with the others. This immediately catches one's eye coming out of the woods. I would expect this meadow to be blooming lushly with wildflowers throughout spring and summer.

At this point the trail is about 150 yards off and parallel to the road that goes to the caretaker's home as it heads into a patch of trees and dense understory dominated by elderberries and buckthorns. The trail drops down through this island of trees and shrubs on its way back to the parking lot at the bottom. A link to other trail systems will become a reality with the building of a 10-foot-wide paved trail and box culvert from the beach facility and out under County Road 41. This project was started in spring 2012.

NEARBY ACTIVITIES

The Minnesota Landscape Arboretum, a living showcase of the state's flora, is only a few miles away. There are hiking trails throughout its grounds, too.

LAKE REBECCA PARK RESERVE 45

IN BRIEF

This expansive park provides good examples of how a forest slowly regains the abandoned agricultural fields of early settlers. The trail circles Lake Rebecca through meadows and younger-growth forests.

DESCRIPTION

Geologically speaking, Lake Rebecca Park Reserve lies on the ground moraine deposited by the Des Moines lobe of the Wisconsin ice age glacial material. The park has rolling countryside that was clear-cut by early settlers for agricultural use. Much of that land continues to revert naturally back to a Big Woods forested composition in what is called "old field" succession. Maple and basswood forests are slowly regaining footholds as this park returns to a more woodsy nature. The Hennepin Regional Park District is still acquiring land for the park. When complete, Lake Rebecca Park Reserve will have more than 2,500 acres. The bike/hike trail offers the best all-around experience at Lake Rebecca.

Head north on the paved trail, where you'll see box elders and open, grassy, rolling hills giving way to overgrown prairielike country as the trail meanders through some of the

KEY AT-A-GLANCE INFORMATION

LENGTH: 6.5 miles

CONFIGURATION: Loop

DIFFICULTY: Easy; gentle rises/ falls in elevation with no strenuous inclines

SCENERY: Woodsy and advanced meadows; few vistas of the lake

EXPOSURE: Mostly full sun; some shade

TRAFFIC: Shared with bicycles; light pedestrian traffic

TRAIL SURFACE: Paved throughout

HIKING TIME: 2.25–3 hours

SEASON: Trails closed November 1–March 31

ACCESS: No fees

MAPS: Available at park headquarters or at threeriversparks.org

FACILITIES: Picnic area with shelter, concessions, restrooms

SPECIAL COMMENTS: Plan time to visit the Trumpeter Swan Restoration Project area.

CONTACT: (763) 694-7860

Directions

Drive west from Minneapolis on US 12 past Maple Plain toward Delano. Just before Delano, turn right (north) on CR 92 and drive about 2 miles to CR 11. Turn left (west), and go 2.5 miles to CR 50 (Town Line Road). Turn right (north), and drive 1.5 miles to the park. Upon entering the park, take a left and go to the far end of the parking lot. The trailhead begins at the extreme north end of the lot.

GPS TRAILHEAD COORDINATES

Latitude   N93° 44.918'

Longitude   W45° 4.399'

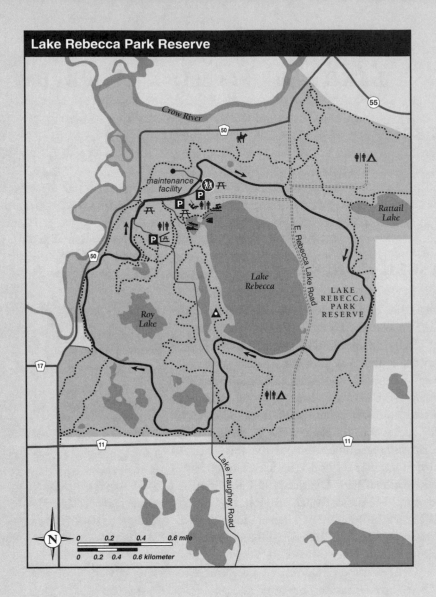

higher elevations in the park. Soon, however, the trail drops into a thicket of maples and basswoods as it continues along a ridge that seems to follow an old river channel. The Crow River is a few hundred yards to your left, but the trail never approaches the river.

You'll come to a short section of split-rail fencing on the left and a subtle overlook onto a small pothole partially visible through the thick understory. Continue along the ridge, which is about 25 feet above the forest floor on your left. The trail then doglegs slightly to the left before continuing on about 0.7 mile to its intersection with Lake Rebecca Road.

However, just before the road, there will be a clearly marked fork in the trail. Take the right fork (the left takes you to Lake Sarah, 0.5 mile to the north), which will lead you toward Lake Rebecca and the interior of the park. You will come up and out of the thicketlike forest area onto a hilly, meadowlike area with sumacs, box elders, and a few scattered cedars. The gravel road intersects the trail just as you reach this opening.

Like others in the park, this meadow represents one of the many stages of the recovery that the park's open areas are making as they slowly return to the forested cover that existed prior to the settlers' presence 150 years ago. You will notice taller trees already making a stand in this meadow. Farther along the hike, meadows in varying stages of regrowth can be compared to each other as this rejuvenation process continues.

The trail slowly climbs for about 0.5 mile to the top of the meadow. At the very top of the climb, check out the elmlike trees on your left. These are actually ironwoods. They tend to be tall and slender, and their leaves are very much like elm leaves except that they are thinner and finer. You will also find sumacs, burr oaks, ashes, and dogwoods—all examples of the types of vegetation gradually encroaching onto the prairie areas.

The trail cuts through a thicket of sumac before dropping down as it meanders along the eastern section of the lake. At about 1.5 miles, you'll come upon a picnic table and the trail will cross over a creek running from Rattail Lake to the east. The trail carves a few big S turns before rising again through a growth of ironwood and a mix of mature maples, burr oaks, and box elders—all in a thick understory.

Soon the trail opens back up to a corridor, a more airy canopy of shorter trees on each side. At about 2.3 miles, this trail again crosses Lake Rebecca Road and drops into stands of maples. As you come out onto marshy lowlands at the southern end of Lake Rebecca, the trail again cuts through more forested areas of box elders and maples.

The trail follows the south end of the lake for about 0.5 mile. Cattails, rushes, and willows are the dominant vegetation in this area—all typical of a Minnesota marsh. At about 3 miles, the trail makes a sharp left away from the lake. You cross an intersection with the bike trail and a spur to the group camp. Stay on the main trail, and as it turns look over your right shoulder to see a small, hidden bay of Lake Rebecca. This is a good birding area for waterfowl, perhaps even a crane or great blue heron.

From here the trail ascends from the lake into another meadow area. Again, check out the encroachment of taller vegetation and trees into this grassland. You'll see saplings of ash and aspen whips mixed with other advancing species. You'll also notice a plantationlike row of trees on the rolling hills above the lake.

The trail drops down to lower elevations once more as it parallels the horse trail along the southern boundary of the park. It climbs again through maples and ironwoods—larger trees than in the last section—and swings north for about 0.5 mile before turning west.

At about 4.1 miles, the trail enters a meadow area, this one with several winding hills and great, open expanses. The trail runs west for about 0.4 mile. At about 4.7 miles along the trail, another picnic table rests beside the edge of yet another marshy area. There is a small parking lot/staging area for the horse trail on the left at about 4.9 miles.

The trail once more heads north, this time following the western boundary of the park. Around mile 6, the trail reconnects with the park road, and the parking lot is about 0.5 mile away.

NEARBY ACTIVITIES

Immediately accessible is the short hiking-only loop to the right of the main entrance. It's only 0.5 mile through a forested area within the park. You are also close to Lake Sarah Regional Park and its recreational amenities.

RUM RIVER CENTRAL REGIONAL PARK

IN BRIEF

One of several hiking opportunities along the popular Rum River, this hike follows a major bend in the river. It also offers a short but scenic hike through central Minnesota river lowlands.

DESCRIPTION

This is primarily a horseback-riding park, but the trails are designated for horses and hikers. There is a separate bike trail, too. Both parallel the river. Start from the north end of the parking lot, and head to the left. This area has marshy lowlands, but soon the trail rises into stands of hardwoods and twists through oaks, basswoods, birches, and even some evergreens. Songbirds seem to be particularly active and vocal in this section, too.

The trail passes through some open areas as it crosses the road near the entrance to the park. From there the trail meanders through oak savanna areas and more trees and marshy spots on its way to the river. About 0.5 mile from the entrance to the park, you will meet up with Rum River and be able to walk along it for nearly 1 mile.

The Rum River flows out of Mille Lacs Lake about 60 road miles to the north. The

KEY AT-A-GLANCE INFORMATION

LENGTH: 3 miles

CONFIGURATION: Loop

DIFFICULTY: Easy; level walking but trail sometimes soft and muddy

SCENERY: Many views of the river, lowlands, and some meadows with wildflowers

EXPOSURE: Shady along the river; sunny in the uplands of meadows

TRAFFIC: Expect weekends to be most active.

TRAIL SURFACE: Earthen; some well churned by horses

HIKING TIME: 1.5–2 hours

SEASON: Some trail sections reserved for skiers in winter

ACCESS: $5 daily vehicle permit; $25 annual county park permit; reciprocity with Washington and Carver County park passes

MAPS: Available at the park or at anokacountyparks.com

FACILITIES: Picnic area with pavilion, restroom, drinking water, playground

SPECIAL COMMENTS: I think it's best to choose this park during drier seasons.

CONTACT: (763) 757-3920

Directions

From Minneapolis, take **US 169 north** to Anoka. In Anoka take **CR 47 north** about 6 miles to 179th Lane Northwest. Turn right and drive for about 1 mile to CR 7. The park entrance is right across the street. Take the park road to the Visitor Contact Station; then follow the road past the horse-trailer parking lot to the next parking lot on the left, about 0.3 mile into the park.

GPS TRAILHEAD COORDINATES

Latitude   N93° 22.677'

Longitude   W45° 17.815'

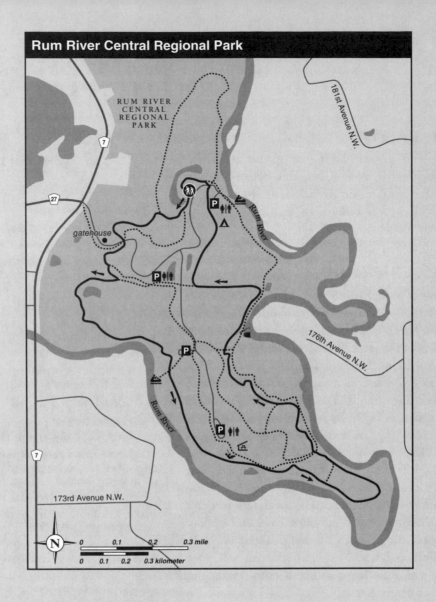

RUM RIVER
CENTRAL
REGIONAL
PARK

181st Avenue N.W.

gatehouse

176th Avenue N.W.

Rum River

173rd Avenue N.W.

N

0   0.1   0.2   0.3 mile

0   0.1   0.2   0.3 kilometer

Rum winds over an additional 40 miles after leaving the park on its way to the Mississippi River. The river forms the southern, eastern, and northern boundaries of this park as it meanders for about 4 miles through this area.

Once walking beside the riverbank, you will soon come to the walk-in canoe-launch area. For the next 0.8 mile or so, the trail meanders along a peninsulalike strip of land, passing through a variety of vegetation common to floodplains as well as some of the higher growth from those wet areas.

The river nearly doubles back on itself at this point along the southern boundary. The banks are lined with box elder and ash trees with a few cottonwoods common to Minnesota's river country.

Following the lead of the river, the trail twists abruptly back along a hairpin turn that heads north. About 120 yards after the trail loops back, you will cross

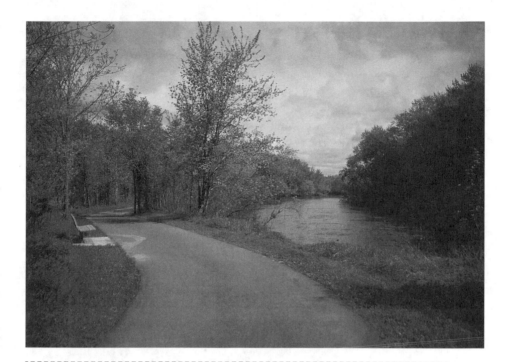

The level bike trail runs along Rum River; the footpath is to the left.

the paved bicycle path. At this point the two trails (bike and horse/hike) parallel each other as they follow the east bank of the river upstream. The bike trail and horse path are separated by a thin corridor of brush and thickets, but there are several places hikers could poke through to get glimpses of the river.

Soon after crossing the bike trail, you'll encounter another horse trail to the left. Stay on a straight course and continue to follow the river. About 0.2 mile farther, you'll come to another horse trail on the left. Again opt for the trail straight ahead.

The trail rises about 30–40 feet as it starts to turn away from the river. At this point you will notice that the oaks and basswoods are quite a bit bigger. The forest is more like upland hardwoods. The basswood, with big heart-shaped leaves, is a dominant species here. It's also called linden when used for landscaping.

You will soon come to an intersection, another junction with the paved bike trail. The hiking trail continues across the paved trail for about 500 feet before taking a sharp turn away from the river and into the heart of the park. The trees are larger here, denser canopies made up of sizable box elders.

Another 500 feet beyond this last intersection, the trail curves sharply to the right and heads back toward the horse trailer parking lot. However, as a hiker, you should turn right about 0.1 mile down this stretch. This will lead you past the canoe campsite and back to the parking lot and trailhead.

NEARBY ACTIVITIES

Visit Rum River North, which is just up the road, and Elm Creek Park Reserve a few minutes south for more hiking possibilities. The town of Anoka offers restaurants and local, small-town shopping. Also consider canoeing along the Rum River; a great half-day paddle is possible from the Rum River North County Park by St. Francis down to this park. There are no canoe rentals or shuttles available, so you'll need to have your own gear and means of getting back to your car.

RUM RIVER NORTH COUNTY PARK 47

IN BRIEF

One of three county parks along the Rum River, this northern extension lies on the east bank of the river, providing excellent views of the water while you pass under a thick canopy of northern hardwoods.

DESCRIPTION

The Rum River is one of those rivers with a northerly feel that are close enough to enjoy with only a short drive from the Twin Cities. I spent many a weekend along its banks as a Boy Scout.

The trail starts at the main pavilion next to the parking lot. Basically the trail follows the river as it forms the boundary for the western edge of this park. Both ends of the trail loop back onto the mail trail to provide about 2 miles of hiking within the park's boundaries.

From the pavilion, hike north along the paved trail that joins the river at a T intersection, and take a right to follow along the riverbank heading upstream. You'll pass by a platform that overlooks the river and presents a nice water's-edge view up- and downstream. The river is not too wide at this point, and the banks are covered in foliage and trees overhanging the water.

Directions ————————————————→

From Minneapolis, drive north on US 169 to Anoka. Take CR 47 north (right) to St. Francis. In St. Francis, turn right onto Ambassador Boulevard and then turn right on Bridge Street. Take the bridge over the Rum River. Take next left after Anoka County Library (on left) onto Rum River Boulevard. Go 500 feet, and take left into park. Turn right after 200 feet, and park in lot next to main pavilion.

i KEY AT-A-GLANCE INFORMATION

LENGTH: 4.4 miles

CONFIGURATION: Elongated figure eight

DIFFICULTY: Very easy; few changes in elevation; smooth trail surface

SCENERY: Trail follows river for most of route through modest overstory of trees

EXPOSURE: Mostly shaded by overstory of trees lining the river

TRAFFIC: Promoted as a multiuse park; lots of activities all year long

TRAIL SURFACE: 1-mile loop is paved; wooded section along arm is packed turf.

HIKING TIME: 1.5–2 hours

SEASON: Year-round; could be very pretty in winter

ACCESS: $5 daily vehicle permit, $25 annual regional park permit; reciprocity with Washington and Carver County park passes

MAPS: Available at the park or at anokacountyparks.com

SPECIAL COMMENTS: Access to this park is right in the city of St. Francis.

CONTACT: (763) 757-3920

GPS TRAILHEAD COORDINATES

Latitude   N93° 21.323'

Longitude   W45° 23.397'

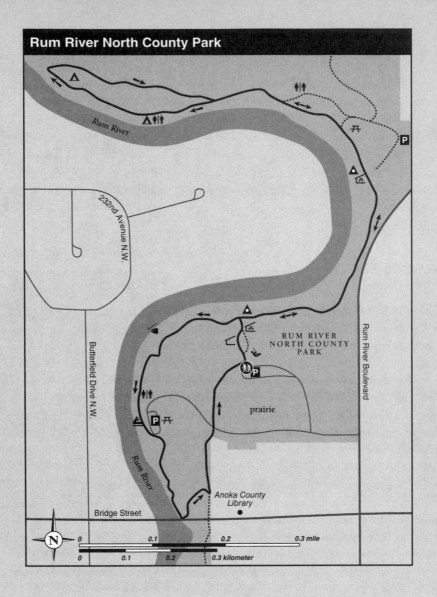

Rum River

232nd Avenue N.W.

Butterfield Drive N.W.

RUM RIVER
NORTH COUNTY
PARK

Rum River Boulevard

prairie

Rum River

Anoka County
Library

Bridge Street

N

| 0 | | 0.1 | | 0.2 | | 0.3 mile |
| 0 | | 0.1 | | 0.2 | | 0.3 kilometer |

Becoming crushed gravel shortly after leaving the center complex of picnic area and parking, the trail meanders through stands of oaks and maples common to this area. Other hardwoods line the bank above the river and along the trail for a few hundred yards until you reach an open, meadowlike area on the right. Here you'll spy another picnic area and pavilion with several sets of tables. The river at this point flows along the base of a fairly steep embankment but always in close proximity to the trail.

On the river side of the trail where it opens to this meadow, you'll find sumacs, oaks, and a few red pines. The trail then swings to the left and drops to very near the river's edge. Notice how the trees change from the upper hardwoods of oaks and maples to the lower floodplain varieties of box elders and silver maples. These are fast-growing trees of much softer wood than their upland neighbors.

Soon the trail splits; this is the intersection for the northern loop. Either fork brings you back to the main trail. Stick to the river's edge by taking the left fork. This trail clings to the river as it passes through a stand of silver maples. Soon you will come to another intersection to the right at the top of this loop. That trail spur leads a few yards out to the canoe camp and take-out site.

As you continue around the loop, you'll move away from the river and soon come upon a marshy area past the trees on the left. Look for some waterbird activity in this area during the spring and early summer. This trail loops back to the main trail and brings you back along the same route, which leads to the starting T intersection up by the first pavilion.

Once you arrive at that T again, keep going straight to reach the southern half of the park. Laid out the same way as the northern section, the trail here follows the river and loops at the end to bring you back through the park.

This end of the trail seems to snake through the woods a bit more than in the northern section, and the rolling nature of it as it dips and climbs the shallow hills makes for a nice undulating walkway along the river. It comes out at a lower parking area and picnic ground. This is a very peaceful, pleasant spot just north of the highway bridge crossing the Rum River in St. Francis.

The trail takes a hard turn to the left at the bridge and goes up to an access point next to the Anoka County Library. To return to the center parking area, head back through the parking lot and take the road out of the lot and up the hill. You will come to a trail intersection on the left that winds through the woods and ends up back at the main pavilion.

A great way to enjoy the park would be to bring a picnic lunch and park at the southern lot. You could then take your lunch and stop over at the canoe take-out area at the extreme northern point for a picnic before heading back down. Or you could leave your basket of goodies at the southern end and hike the entire loop before having a picnic right along the riverbank at the south end of the park. Either option offers a good way to enjoy this short stretch of the Rum River.

NEARBY ACTIVITIES

Other hikes are farther north, so your planning may include this hike at the start or end of a day's hiking along these northern Twin Cities routes.

48 SAND DUNES STATE FOREST,
Ann Lake

KEY AT-A-GLANCE INFORMATION

LENGTH: 2 miles

CONFIGURATION: Elongated loop

DIFFICULTY: Moderate to easy throughout with some short but steep inclines

SCENERY: Plantations of white and red pine; oak-covered sandy ridges

EXPOSURE: Mixed full sun and dense shade within the plantations

TRAFFIC: Trail loops through less-developed, lower-traffic northern area of park

TRAIL SURFACE: Sandy and hard-packed earthen trails throughout

HIKING TIME: 1 hour

SEASON: Year-round; the pines are especially beautiful after a snowfall.

ACCESS: No fees

MAPS: Available at kiosk on-site (Sand Dunes State Forest Trail Map)

FACILITIES: Campground, outhouse, picnic area, drinking water, beach, and swimming area

SPECIAL COMMENTS: The sand country is quite different from the bedrock glaciated areas farther east and south; stands of pines offer a pleasant alternative to predominantly hardwood forests.

CONTACT: (768) 878-2325 or www.dnr.state.mn.us/state_forests/sft00045

GPS TRAILHEAD COORDINATES

Latitude   N93° 41.600'
Longitude   W45° 25.599'

IN BRIEF

One of many in the Sand Dunes State Forest, this hiker-only trail wanders through Bob Dunn Recreation Area. It highlights white and red pine plantations and offers a good example of Minnesota's northern sandy soil country.

DESCRIPTION

This hike lies in the midst of a greater natural/recreational area made up of the Sherburne National Wildlife Refuge, the Sand Dunes State Forest, and the Uncas Dunes Scientific and Natural Area. Multipurpose trails weave through the area. This representative hike in the Bob Dunn Recreation Area showcases the region's more than 3 miles of earthen paths.

Start at the end of the parking lot by the picnic area. The trailhead is to the right, across the road. The lake is just a few steps farther on. Head up the trail into an area forested with oak, spruce, and red pine. The trail immediately climbs a small sandy knoll before taking a sharp right about 50 yards from the trailhead. This is a stretch of the Yellow Trail. You're on the correct path if you come to an old hand-operated water pump on your left.

These sandy areas tend to produce solid stands of oaks. The trail will meander through groves that combine red and pin oaks. Spruce

----

Directions

Take US 169 north from Minneapolis to Zimmerman, Minnesota. Take CR 4 west (left) 4.5 miles past CR 15 to 168th Street. Take a left, and go 0.2 mile to Dunes Forest Road. Turn right following the sign to Ann Lake. Drive 0.6 mile to the entrance of Bob Dunn Recreation Area on the left. Follow the road to the parking lot and picnic area.

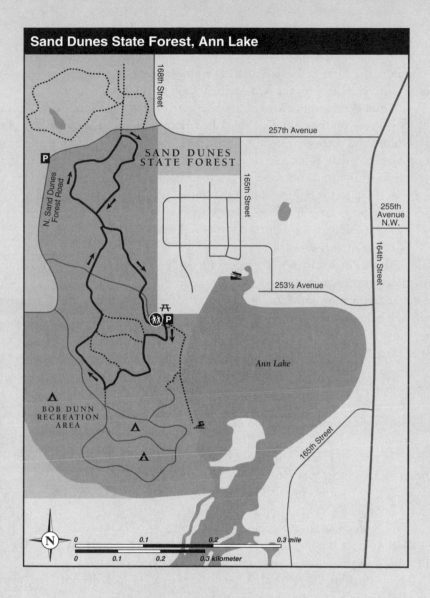

seedlings, also part of the sandy soil ecology, have sprouted throughout this park. Past the water pump, these seedlings, some 3–4 feet tall, dominate the understory.

As you top the hill, you'll see the fire tower on your left. You can't climb it, but vistas reveal the surrounding area over the tops of the oaks below. You'll pass two intersections: the other end of the Yellow Loop and the beginning of the Orange Loop. Stay to the left past these two intersections. You will then be on the back half of the Orange Loop. This particular hike takes a clockwise path around the outer loops of the interconnecting color-coded trails.

Just past the fire tower, the trail forks. The sandy path on the left drops down to a campsite, while the one to the right descends about 50 feet in elevation to continue the Orange Loop. At the bottom of the hill, you will arrive at yet another intersection, with the Red Loop. Take it to the left.

The trail climbs uphill toward a white-pine plantation. Notice a sign identifying poison ivy on the right. The short Red Loop follows the topography of the park around and through a stand of jack pines. Jack pines are often seen sprouting up after forest fires because their seed coat needs high temperatures to open. This length of the trail cuts close to the road before looping back around to the main trail. Keep to the right, and take the trail as it climbs up into a stand of white pines. White pines have five long, somewhat fine needles in a cluster as well as a smoother, grayish bark—as opposed to the red, scaly bark of the red pine.

As this trail cuts through the stand of white pines, notice the profusion of white pine seedlings scattered like weeds throughout the forest floor. This prolific growth of pines prompted successful plantation development in the 1940s, when the Great Depression saw farming in this sandy-soiled region suffer. Plantations may have helped stabilize the soil, which otherwise would have blown away. To date, more than 2,400 acres of tree plantations have been established in the Sand Dunes State Forest. The majority of these grow pines, as on this trail.

A small cluster of jack pine and a small aspen stand line the trail after the white pine plantation. Just beyond lie an open meadow area and yet another trail intersection. This is the Orange Loop again; take the turn to the left. Now the trail rises in elevation to stands of older, more mature oaks. You will also see a plantation of red pine. Do you notice the difference between these and the earlier whites? If not, you have a second chance. The trail next dips down into still another white pine plantation before coming up on a ridge.

About 200 yards beyond the intersection that brought you back onto the Orange Loop, the Orange Loop veers back to your right. Continue straight; this is the Yellow Loop again. Another 0.1 mile, and you will cross over County Road 254. You are now heading into the northern half of the recreation area. Another 0.15 mile, and you will encounter yet another trail intersection.

This is the Blue Loop, which is a 0.8-mile route through the northern quarter of the Bob Dunn Recreation Area. It continues its serpentine way up and down the sandy hills through varied forest types before coming back on itself. A left at the intersection continues through more mature oaks on the ridge. Again you will see more small white pines gaining a foothold on the ridge. The trail cuts sharply to the right as it passes very near the park boundary. Soon the trail meets up with the main park entrance road and leads back to the parking lot where you began.

NEARBY ACTIVITIES

The Ann Lake trail skirts the western edge of the lake. The southern portion is marshy, a good bird-viewing area. Also, at the north end of the park, is another 0.5-mile loop, the Green Loop. For those seeking still more hiking options, corridors beyond the Blue Loop link it to the North Orock Trail within Sand Dunes State Forest. These are multiuse trails open to hiking and snowmobiling.

SHERBURNE NATIONAL WILDLIFE REFUGE, Prairie's Edge Trail

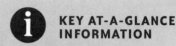

49

IN BRIEF

This is designated as a driving tour, but there is too much to see—so take to foot and enjoy a hike through excellent marshes along the prairie's edge. You'll find it a superb bird-watching tour.

DESCRIPTION

While Prairie's Edge describes the overall topography and terrain characteristics of this hiking area, Marsh's Edge would seem a more appropriate name for the immediate and sur-rounding natural experience one gets from hiking this area. Although this is called a driv-ing trail, there is much too much to observe along these 7.3 miles to chance missing any of it by driving, even at 5–7 mph. The entire marsh community is more easily viewed with-out the drone of a car's engine or the grinding of tires over its gravel surface.

The Sherburne National Wildlife Refuge (NWR) publishes a bird list featuring more than 230 species common or transient to the refuge. If you are a birder and a hiker, this place will reward you several times over. Make sure you bring your binoculars on this hike.

Before starting, take a quick look from the observation deck; then head east along

KEY AT-A-GLANCE INFORMATION

LENGTH: 7.3 miles

CONFIGURATION: Loop with two short side-spur options

DIFFICULTY: Level; very easy

SCENERY: Open meadows and marshes with a few scattered islands of trees

EXPOSURE: Mostly full sun; some shade

TRAFFIC: Occasional vehicle and bike traffic but probably not ever too crowded

TRAIL SURFACE: Hard-packed gravel roadway

HIKING TIME: 2.5–3 hours

SEASON: April–October

ACCESS: No fees

MAPS: Available in box inside entrance or at fws.gov/midwest /sherburne/prairie.htm

FACILITIES: None

SPECIAL COMMENTS: Use caution here when sharing the road with vehicles.

CONTACT: (763) 389-3323

Directions

Go north from Minneapolis on US 169 to Zimmerman. Turn west (left) onto CR 4/261st Avenue (also signed as Freemont Avenue). Go west about 7.5 miles to CR 5. Turn north (right), and go about 1.25 miles to entrance to refuge on right. Park in small lot immediately on your left about 0.25 mile from the entrance near the observation station and a handicapped-accessible trail.

GPS TRAILHEAD COORDINATES

Latitude   N93° 43.865'

Longitude   W45° 27.955'

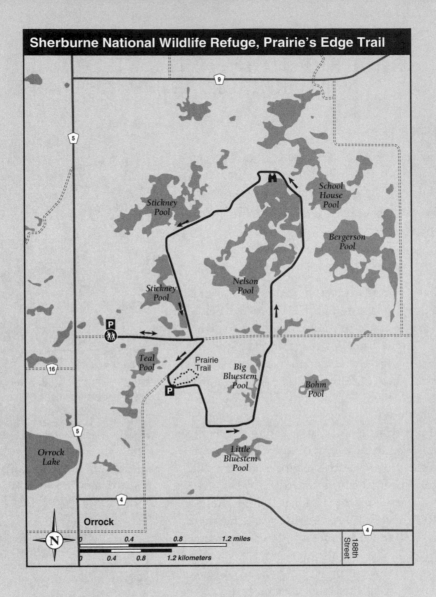

the entrance road. The first 0.75 mile brings you straight into the heart of the Sherburne NWR. About 0.5 mile from the observation area is a small pond on the right called Teal Pool. It and 23 other pools throughout the park have been developed from naturally occurring, uncontrolled pools, and their water levels are regulated to create a number of different wetland types.

The prairie/marshland mix preserved in this park is a prime example of what these prairie-bordering areas were like as transition zones between the forested areas of the eastern United States and those of the tall-grass prairies of Minnesota and beyond. Many of the wild critters and birds indigenous to this area today are the same species that were found here more than 150 years ago—just as the settlers of this region found them. In all, the refuge covers more than 30,000 acres in a mosaic of oak savanna, wetlands, and the Big Woods habitat.

The road around the Prairie's Edge directs visitors counterclockwise around the loop, so don't take the intersection on your left near the end of this first straightaway road. Instead, go straight another 0.2 mile, and follow the road as it turns sharply to the right. You are now on the loop that will continue for another 6 miles.

Teal Pool will be on your right as you climb a bit into the higher prairie country. As the road cuts back to the left, a short side trail on the left, called the Prairie Trail, makes a short, 0.4-mile loop through typical tall-grass meadow and prairie vegetation. About 0.3 mile beyond the Prairie Trail, the road swings right again to lead through the first of many marshy areas. You will also cross over one of the many drainage canals used to regulate the water in all the pools throughout the refuge.

Crossing this marsh grass area, the trail cuts left again and passes along Little Bluestem Pool. Stop at the observation area at the middle point of the pool, and try to spot some of the waterbirds and shore species that frequent the park. Using your binoculars, inspect the edges of the rushes right at the waterline for such species as little green herons and sora rails—otherwise very hard to see against the backdrop of rushes.

Past this lookout 0.25 mile, the road turns north and, for the next 1.5 miles, cuts along the edge of several pools including the many ponds of Big Bluestem Pool on the left. You may have the best luck spotting critters by walking a few yards and then stopping for a few moments and studying any movements you see. Along this entire roadway, signs with black symbols display songbirds and other wildlife that may be seen in the immediate vicinity.

About 0.5 mile past the end of Big Bluestem Pool, the road swings slightly to the right to pass between two of the refuge's biggest pools—Bergerson Pool on the right and Nelson Pool on the left. Bergerson measures nearly 1 mile across. As the roadway heads north it comes right alongside Nelson Pool to skirt its shoreline for the next 0.7 mile or more.

The road turns northwest and then due west at the upper end of School House Pool. At the northwest tip of the pool is yet another observation area. If you look due south a few hundred yards, you should see a large dead tree with an eagle's nest at its top. If there are too many people present to get a good view, don't worry; a closer viewing point is available farther along the trail, just after it makes a 90-degree turn to the left (south). A few hundred yards farther, it starts to turn again. On the left is the pool, and a few thin spots in the bordering trees should allow you to get a good look at the nest.

The trail now turns to the southwest, where you will come upon a sample of the woodlands associated with the oak savanna habitat. Look for songbirds in this area. Although it's a common nester in the park, I spotted my first rose-breasted grosbeak in this area during my hike. About 0.5 mile from the bend in the road where you viewed the eagle's nest through the trees, there is another trail spur called the Woodland Trail. This 0.5-mile trail takes you through one of the woodland islands common to this oak savanna country.

The next 0.5 mile skirts along yet another pool, this one unnamed on the map. The trail then drops south again and passes Stickney Pool. The next 0.6 mile takes you right along its edge, too. By now you should be pretty good at detecting all the creatures hiding among the rushes.

When the road comes to a T intersection, this marks the end of the Prairie's Edge loop. A right takes you back to the first observation area and your car.

NEARBY ACTIVITIES

The Sherburne NWR has two other hiking options: the Mahnomen Trails, with about 2.6 miles of trails, and the Blue Hill Trail, with a trail network of more than 5 miles. Both of these are north of the Prairie's Edge trail system and offer more upland features and critters. These trails are especially good to hike during the spring and fall migrations, when the woodland songbirds are passing through.

You might also want to visit Ann Lake/Sand Dunes just a few miles south of the refuge.

SNAIL LAKE 50

IN BRIEF

While Vadnais Lake gets top billing, a trail system south of Snail Lake is the notable hiking attraction in this multilake region of northeast St. Paul. The primitive marshy area right in the backyard of moderately priced homes provides an appealing transition between the city and Minnesota's lakes and marshes.

DESCRIPTION

Snail Lake and Vadnais Lake share the spotlight for a multiple-lake regional park that is just outside the freeway loop around northern St. Paul. There are several trail options to consider, including a great sampler that begins in the parking lot of the Snail Lake Regional Park.

From the lot, take the paved bike/hike trail that leads under Snail Lake Boulevard via a tunnel, or walk across the street from the entrance to hook up with the same trail. The paths immediately fork—take the right fork and head into the wooded area away from the marshy lowlands on your left. This trail heads slightly uphill through a scattering of oaks and maples. It's fairly open, with older oaks sprinkled about. The path continues on to what first appears to be a knoll, but as you walk deeper into the wooded area you learn that it's a knob on the side of the slope that drops

---

Directions

From Minneapolis, go north on I-35 West to I-694. Go east about 3 miles to Exit 43B (Victoria Street). Go north (left) to Snail Lake Boulevard. From St. Paul, take I-35 East to I-694, and head west about 3.5 miles to Exit 43B. Turn right (east), and go about 0.7 mile to park entrance on left (just past Mackubin Street).

KEY AT-A-GLANCE INFORMATION

LENGTH: 3.2 miles

CONFIGURATION: Barbell shape

DIFFICULTY: Easy to moderate with a few steep areas

SCENERY: Pleasantly woodsy with rolling hills, marshy transition zones, and open marsh in southern half

EXPOSURE: Northern half is shaded; southern half is exposed.

TRAFFIC: Eastern trail follows backyard boundary of homes, but southern marsh and northern woods areas offer solitude

TRAIL SURFACE: Paved throughout

HIKING TIME: 1.5–1.75 hours

SEASON: Year-round; snowshoeing is popular here in winter.

ACCESS: No fees

MAPS: Intersections are marked; maps at www.co.ramsey.mn.us /parks/parks/snaillake.htm

FACILITIES: Playground, picnic area, restrooms, drinking water

SPECIAL COMMENTS: Marsh areas are left in their natural state, so this should be a good bird-watching park in spring and summer. It offers a good sense of a northern woods, even with houses visible right from the trail, and pedestrian underpasses beneath roadways.

CONTACT: (651) 748-2500

GPS TRAILHEAD COORDINATES

Latitude   N93° 7.379'

Longitude   W45° 4.041'

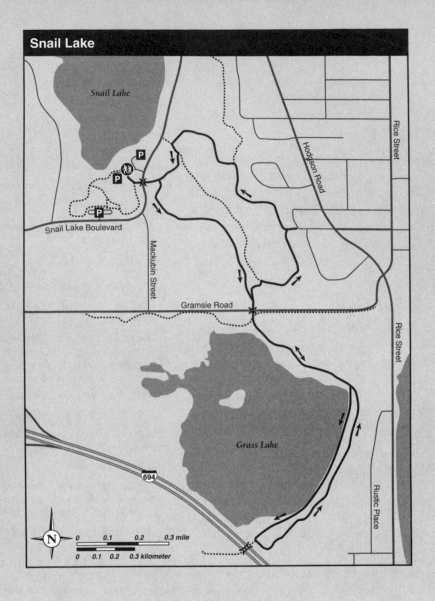

Snail Lake

Hodgson Road

Rice Street

P

Snail Lake Boulevard

Mackubin Street

Gramsie Road

Rice Street

Grass Lake

694

Rustic Place

0   0.1   0.2   0.3 mile

0   0.1   0.2   0.3 kilometer

N

down from the road and forms the sides of the basin containing the marshy areas to the south.

The trail does become hillier, with red and white oaks as the dominant trees in the immediate area with a dense understory beneath. A few minor trails spur off this main trail. Their presence is made known only by modest hard-packed earthen paths that veer off as unannounced side trails. The ones on the left probably link up with the trails that cut down the center of the park.

Serpentine and hilly, the trail offers moderately easy hiking through dense but not imposing woodlands. About a quarter of the way down the first loop, you'll cross under a power line. There is a swath cut to the pond for a glimpse of what lies beyond the trees.

Like other parks surrounded by highways, this one has the sound of traffic woven into it. It's best to dwell not on the noise but on the fact that you can walk through trees rather than alongside fast-moving cars on a freeway.

As you near the southern end of the Snail Lake loop of trails, you'll come through a short corridor of young aspen. As you exit it, Gramsie Road appears in the background. A stand of cedar trees flanks the hill on the left overlooking a grassy meadow area through which the trail extends before going under the road to continue along the east side of Grass Lake. For those desiring only a short hike, keep on the paved path instead of taking the trail to the tunnel beneath Gramsie, and continue back along the trail as it curves back to the north. About 0.5 mile farther, a trail to the left will take you back to Snail Lake Boulevard and back over to the parking lot. Otherwise, head for the tunnel for the remaining 2 miles of the hike.

The trail forks shortly after the tunnel. Follow the hiking trail to the left alongside Grass Lake. At the bottom of the loop, you'll come to the intersection with the bike trail. The bike path to the right joins up with a regional bike corridor, but you want to take a left and head back to the tunnel.

When you have returned to the pedestrian/bike underpass, turn right, and after about 80 yards the trail forks. The right fork heads to the east and follows the eastern side of the marsh, while the left fork stays along the bike trail that cuts down the center of the park. Take the right fork for a slightly longer walk, and one that stays closer to the edge of the marshy area.

This pathway also follows the backyard property lines of houses adjacent to the trail. Aspens, box elders, and some maples and hazel brush line this walkway, which is about 40 feet from the marshy shoreline.

About three-fourths of the way around the marshy area, there are more islands and outcrops of alders, willows, and shrublike trees. Alders are like little birch trees, as their leaves and catkins have the same shape.

The marsh is long and narrow with cottonwoods at its northern end. More houses skirt the perimeter just before the trail turns around and returns to its origin. If taken, another fork at the northeastern end of the lake leads you north to the intersection of the trail with County Road 96. There you are directed to more hiking along a regional trail. Otherwise, take the trail fork to the left. The trail swings back around into a hilly area before descending the back side of that small marsh you passed on your way in. You can take the underpass tunnel back to the parking lot.

NEARBY ACTIVITIES

The Vadnais–Snail Lake Regional Park, offering more trails, lies about a mile east of Snail Lake.

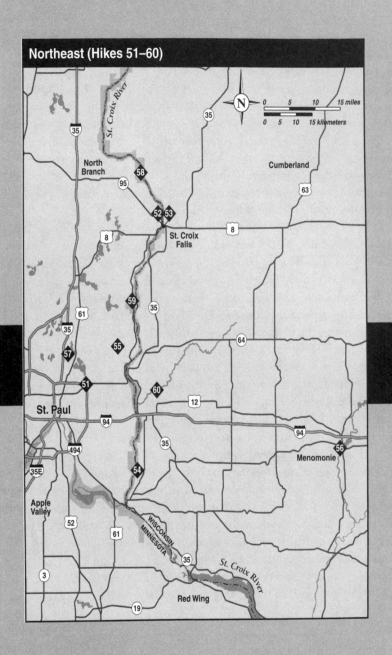

Northeast (Hikes 51–60)

North Branch

Cumberland

St. Croix Falls

St. Paul

Menomonie

Apple Valley

WISCONSIN

MINNESOTA

Red Wing

St. Croix River

0 5 10 15 miles
0 5 10 15 kilometers

NORTHEAST

51 GATEWAY STATE TRAIL

KEY AT-A-GLANCE INFORMATION

LENGTH: 9.7 miles (one way)

CONFIGURATION: Point to point

DIFFICULTY: Easy

SCENERY: Countryside, both natural and agricultural; a few lakes

EXPOSURE: Open sun and shady corridors throughout

TRAFFIC: Light hiking, with heavy use by bicyclists

TRAIL SURFACE: Paved throughout

HIKING TIME: 3–4 hours

SEASON: Year-round

ACCESS: Minnesota State Park fee system: $5 daily, $25 annual permit, $12 annual permit for disabled individuals

MAPS: At trailheads or online at www.dnr.state.mn.us/state_trails/gateway

FACILITIES: None along trail; restrooms, drinking water, and interpretive information at north end; several stores near southern terminus of this hike

SPECIAL COMMENTS: This woodsy, pastoral corridor takes you immediately from the sights and sounds of a major freeway intersection to the bucolic solitude of eastern Minnesota farm country—with pockets of nature tossed in for your appreciation and enjoyment.

CONTACT: (651) 296-6157

GPS TRAILHEAD COORDINATES

Latitude   N93° 57.778'

Longitude   W45° 1.589'

IN BRIEF

The Gateway State Trail is a section of the old Soo railway bed, which has been converted into a multiuse trail that cuts through miles of urban, suburban, and rural areas. This well-maintained paved trail affords a wide variety of nonmotorized traffic miles and miles of open countryside, small woodlots and lakes, and small clusters of farm and pasture land.

DESCRIPTION

The country setting is the charm of the northern half of the Gateway State Trail, which begins in the residential section of Lake Phalen in St. Paul. The hike ends just north of Stillwater at Pine Point Regional Park. The "city" half of this 18.3-mile-long trail joins up with other St. Paul trail systems. It's not until you get past the swarm of traffic at the intersection of I-694 and MN 36 in the suburbs east of St. Paul that you really get to see the true character of this trail.

Once you leave the parking lot on your 9.7-mile hike northeastward, the only urban structures you'll see except for a few road crossings are the tunnels beneath both highways during the first 0.5 mile of this hike. In fact, since this hike starts at the trail's halfway

----

Directions

The trailhead for this hike is located off Hadley Avenue in Oakdale. From I-35 East, go east on MN 36 (Exit 111). Turn right onto Hadley Avenue just before the exit ramp onto I-694 South. Go a quarter of a block to 55th Street North, and turn left (east). Continue for 0.5 mile to the parking-lot entrance on the right. From I-694, take Exit 52 to west MN 36. Turn left (south) onto Hadley Avenue just west of the intersection of I-694 and MN 36.

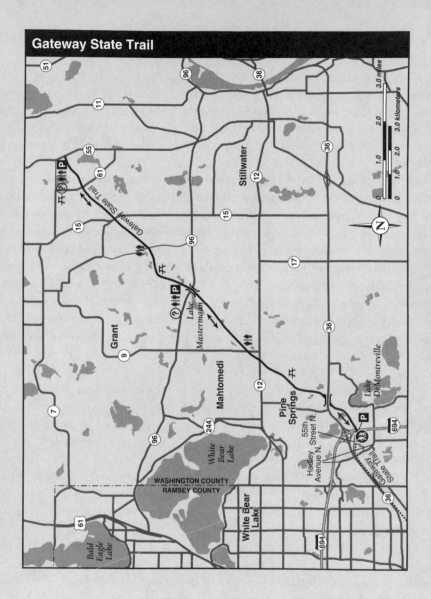

point, the first milepost you'll encounter just beyond the I-694 underpass is actually number 9.

From the parking lot, the trail immediately takes you beneath the drone of traffic and into a wooded, parklike area between the two highway intersections. This 0.5-mile-long segment also has trail spurs leading off to other, shorter loops that head south toward Lake De Montreville. You know you have left the urban portion of this hike by milepost 9 when the horseback-riding trail begins to parallel the paved trail for the entire length northeastward to Washington County's Pine Point Regional Park.

Continuing past the cavernous tunnel under MN 36 leads you immediately onto a tree-lined corridor that is pretty much consistent for nearly all of the next

10 miles. The wooded thicket of cherry, ash, oak, and box elder trees before the tunnel now opens onto a small pond, marshy area, and rail fence on the north (left) side of the trail. Wildflowers abound where the pavement ends. This section has a river-bottomlands feel to it (with box elders and aspens)—and you can appreciate this even more if you realize that downtown St. Paul is less than 10 miles away.

Approaching milepost 10, the surroundings become wetlands with cattails growing just off the trail in the foreground and grassy meadows in the distance. The tree canopy opens up at this point, allowing more sunlight to penetrate down to the trail. By milepost 11, the marshy area is reduced to a few cattails along the south edge that quickly give way to an expansive, open savannalike area of hills.

At about milepost 11.5, you'll reach a shady area with a kiosk and a bench, and then a double intersection: first with 75th Street/County Road 12 and about 100 yards farther with Jamaica Avenue. This is one of several points along the way where you could leave your car and access the trail in either direction. From this point northward, the trail is separated from a gravel roadway by only about a dozen feet of shrubbery—it could get very dusty on a hot, dry summer day along here.

Aspens, red and white oaks, and 20-foot-tall sumacs stand sentry over the corridor in this section before you reach yet another intersection around mile 12.7. This is the 84th and Jewell intersection, well defined by the power line overhead. Here, tall aspens and oaks continue to dominate the scenery.

Milepost 13 brings a bench alongside the trail. You can enjoy the pond on the south side and a more mature forest dominated by big oaks. Soon after passing this marker, the trail becomes a series of modest but definitely noticeable hills and dips for several yards—breaking up the monotony of an otherwise straight and level trail.

Just past this series of bumps, check out a narrow cut through the trees angling off to the right from the trail. Notice the slightly raised bed in view through the woods—that's likely a spur of the original railroad bed.

Shortly thereafter, you'll approach the intersection and overpass at MN 96. Lake Masterman is on the left but obstructed from view by the cutbank above the trail and the dense understory. Here, about halfway from the midtrail starting point at I-694 and Pine Point Regional Park, is yet another point where you can access the trail for a shorter hiking segment.

Another bench sits at milepost 14. There may be increased horseback-riding activity in this area because you are within a mile of a horse-trailer parking/staging area at milepost 15.

At Lansing Avenue, you'll find a clearing with a picnic table and an outhouse. This is before a long 0.5- to 0.75-mile straight-as-an-arrow corridor. The trail then takes a slight jog right, where it crosses a private driveway. Check out the red pines and cedars along the trail just before your next intersection, which is Manning Avenue (a new bridge span was erected here in November 2011).

You are now within a couple of miles of the western boundary of Pine Point Regional Park. From here to the park is a patchwork of meadows, woodlots, and farmland. The next highway to cross is CR 61, which runs along the western border of the regional park. Once inside the park, you'll find an interwoven network of trails. See the listing for Pine Point Regional Park on page 234 for details on the hiking opportunities there.

NEARBY ACTIVITIES

Beyond either end of the trail are more trail-system connections. Pine Point Regional Park is only about 4 miles north of the river town of Stillwater, and a bit farther from William O'Brien State Park to the north. Also, you are only a few minutes away from the scenic St. Croix River.

52 INTERSTATE STATE PARK, MINNESOTA

KEY AT-A-GLANCE INFORMATION

LENGTH: 0.3 mile along trails in potholes section; 3.8 miles along river and railroad bed; total of 4.1 miles

CONFIGURATION: Loop with spurs

DIFFICULTY: Mostly easy or moderate, with rugged sections along river

SCENERY: Great geologic features and fantastic views of the river

EXPOSURE: Mostly sun; some shade

TRAFFIC: Potholes always attract visitors and even rock-climbing classes; trails used more by campers

TRAIL SURFACE: Some constructed walkways at potholes; earthen trails with exposed roots and rocks

HIKING TIME: 2–3 hours, including time wandering potholes

SEASON: Mostly summer; hazardous in most areas in winter

ACCESS: Potholes: Daily, 8 a.m.–10 p.m. Minnesota State Park fee system: $5 daily, $25 annual permit, $12 annual permit for disabled individuals

MAPS: At park or at www.dnr.state .mn.us/state_parks/interstate

FACILITIES: Restrooms, visitor center/gift shop, drinking water at potholes, boat launch, campground

SPECIAL COMMENTS: Minnesota side of park offers more potholes in a small area and longer hike on river.

CONTACT: (651) 465-5711

GPS TRAILHEAD COORDINATES

Latitude   N92° 39.077'

Longitude W45° 23.997'

IN BRIEF

Walk along expansive river bluffs, a former railroad grade, and one of the world's largest glacial potholes in the Minnesota section of this century-old interstate park. Vistas of the St. Croix valley and environs round out the sights that complement the activities found across the river.

DESCRIPTION

Though Interstate State Park is now protected, at one time this and the surrounding areas provided a valuable resource for the logging industry. With vast tracks of white pine to the north and a wide river to float them down, the logging industry soon proved to be an economic boon to Minnesota and neighboring Wisconsin. As Taylors Falls and the surrounding area became increasingly popular with visitors, many people started building in the Dalles section of the St. Croix valley. Recognizing that the beauty and unspoiled nature of the land was threatened with continual development, a bill was introduced and passed in 1894 authorizing the state to work with Wisconsin to acquire land along the river. More than 1,600 acres were set aside between the two states, and Interstate State Park became the first interstate park in the country.

Directions

From Minneapolis, take I-35 West north; from St. Paul, take I-35 East or US 61 to Forest Lake. At Forest Lake, take US 8 toward Taylors Falls. At the intersection with MN 95, turn left (north) to Taylors Falls. At the intersection just as you are turning right to cross over the bridge into Wisconsin, take a sharp right into the potholes area of Minnesota's Interstate State Park parking lot.

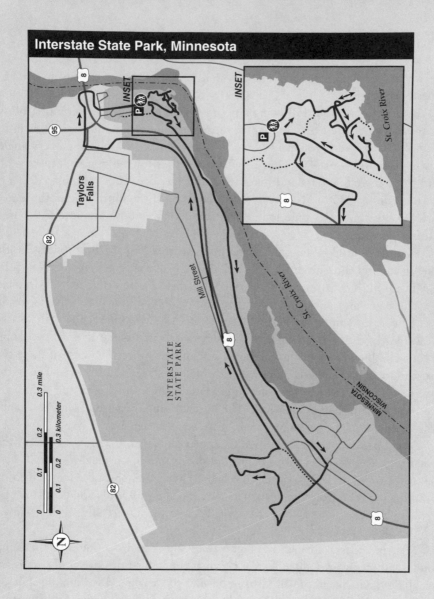

Interstate State Park, Minnesota

Before you start, stop in at the visitor center right at the entrance to the parking lot and see the small museum. When you are ready, begin at the paved pathway beyond the state park office and visitor center at the opposite end of the parking lot from the museum.

The first part of this hike explores the park's amazing potholes. One of these potholes, the Bottomless Pit, is said to be the deepest explored glacial pothole in the world. The route from the visitor center begins just beyond the building and leads down a paved pathway over basalt layers laid down more than 11 billion years ago. You can see the force of erosion from sand and boulders churning in the flowing water. Smooth and wavy formations and myriad potholes ground into the hard rock all attest to the power and persistence of time.

Don't worry about following any prescribed hike (though certainly follow the route I've plotted on the map if you want guidance), and instead, wander around this area until you are satisfied you've seen everything from every angle. This is more like a pre-hike, but it will be worth it for the opportunity to walk amid these huge boulders and outcrops and to get occasional glimpses down to the river and across to Wisconsin from the edge of the bluff. The pothole network is only about 0.3 mile long, but meandering could add another 0.1 mile to this segment.

Part of the trail is self-guided and takes visitors past the Bottomless Pit, the Bake Oven, and the Cauldron. There is a tight L-shaped crack in the rock called the Squeeze. It'll confirm whether or not that diet of yours is actually working.

There are also two spur trails that lead to observation platforms above the river. During the summer, you should see canoeists and kayakers plying the waters below. One of the observation decks is immediately across the river from a popular rock-climbing face on the Wisconsin side of the Dalles. The first of these two observation platforms also allows you to look upstream and down. This right-angle bend in the river is the result of glaciated waters flowing in and then being diverted by a fault line in the basalt. The water, taking the path of least resistance, turns sharply to the right to form this acute bend in the river.

After spending time at the potholes, you embark on a 2.75-mile loop that leads to the Minnesota state campground downstream. To reach this trail, head back toward the parking lot using the main, paved trail and take the trail to the left across the road from the drinking fountain. The trail leads you up a short but steep climb to the highway before cutting back to the left to parallel the roadway atop the slope above the river.

The trail passes through the highway overlook and continues to the campground and picnic area about 1 mile downstream. This primitive trail climbs and dips along the banks of the St. Croix—be sure to wear good scrambling shoes.

At about 0.75 mile from the trailhead, just before you approach the campgrounds, you will come to a fork in the trail. The left fork takes you through the campgrounds, but you want the right fork, which continues past the campground to the information office at the campground entrance.

To the left of the office is a trail spur that heads up to and under the highway via a 6-foot-tall concrete tunnel. Immediately afterward, you'll come to a T intersection. Continue to the left, and follow the signs to the ancient waterfall along the 1-mile Sandstone Bluffs Trail. This trail heads past the massive footings from the old train tracks and up the valley to an "extinct" waterfall. It then climbs the bluff, passes two observation points, and drops back down to join the Railroad Trail. If you don't want the extra 1-mile climb, turn right at the T and follow the Railroad Trail back to town.

The railroad came to Taylors Falls around 1880, long after it had developed as a popular tourist retreat and well into the establishment of the lumber industry that took millions of board feet of white pine out of the area.

This is a straight shot, as railroad rights-of-way tend to be. It's a tree-lined corridor through maples, oaks, and upland hardwood understory. The trail ends at a parking lot behind the Taylors Falls Community Center, a modest white-sided building a few blocks from the pothole section of the park. Continue out to the street. A small schoolhouse, Minnesota's oldest standing schoolhouse, will be on your left as you head to the right down to the next street intersection.

Take a right again, and cross Bench Street, the main street feeding into downtown from the highway on the right. Then head to the left of the entrance onto the bridge. The pathway takes you under the bridge to the right and back up to the entrance to the parking lot at the potholes.

NEARBY ACTIVITIES

Wisconsin's side of the park awaits, and Taylors Falls is a cool tourist town. Riverboat tours depart throughout the day during the summer, and many outfitters in the area rent canoes and gear for paddling on the St. Croix.

53 INTERSTATE STATE PARK, WISCONSIN

KEY AT-A-GLANCE INFORMATION

LENGTH: 4.6 miles

CONFIGURATION: Irregular figure eight with one out-and-back spur

DIFFICULTY: Easy to moderate; some steep grades; uneven footing

SCENERY: Breathtaking vistas and sheer cliff overlooks

EXPOSURE: Sunny along Dalles; shady in maple forests behind bluffs

TRAFFIC: Very popular day destination; hosts rock climbers in summer

TRAIL SURFACE: Uneven earthen path with exposed boulders and roots; narrow and hilly in some areas

HIKING TIME: 2–3 hours

SEASON: Early spring–late fall; slippery and hazardous in winter

ACCESS: $7 daily for Wisconsin residents, $10 out-of-state; $25 annual pass for Wisconsin residents, $35 annual out-of-state

MAPS: At park office at entrance and at www.dnr.state.wi.us/org/land/parks/specific/interstate

FACILITIES: Amphitheater, fishing pier, camping, and interpretive center in park; picnic area, shelter, bathhouse, restrooms, showers, and swimming at Lake O' the Dalles

SPECIAL COMMENTS: More trails than the Minnesota side; bring camera.

CONTACT: (715) 483-3747

GPS TRAILHEAD COORDINATES

Latitude   N92° 38.847'

Longitude   W45° 24.009'

IN BRIEF

Hike through sections of the United States' oldest interstate park, exploring the many billion-year-old geological formations scattered along the trail. This hike complements the interstate hike in Minnesota, offering excellent views of the St. Croix River and 23-acre Lake O' the Dalles.

DESCRIPTION

The Interstate State Park hike on the Wisconsin side begins at the second right after passing the park entrance. The sign at the intersection says NORTH CAMP GROUND. Turn immediately to the left into one of the few spaces in front of the pine trees.

Interstate State Park is part of the National Ice Age Reserve—nine units stretching from Lake Michigan to the St. Croix valley. It's an area rich in geological evidence of the ice age 10,000 years ago that covered most of the upper Midwest in mile-thick ice. The one exception is this area of Wisconsin that was spared the last ice advance. The Dalles of the St. Croix is a spectacular reminder of this period.

The modest parking area for the Pothole Trail is the starting point for a series of looped

---

Directions

From Minneapolis, take I-35 West north; from St. Paul, take I-35 East or US 61 to Forest Lake. Take US 8 toward Taylors Falls. Continue across the bridge into Wisconsin, and go uphill to WI 35 and take a right at the sign to Interstate State Park. Continue south to the park entrance. Stay on the park road to the second right. Park in the spaces adjacent to the intersection with North Camp Ground Road.

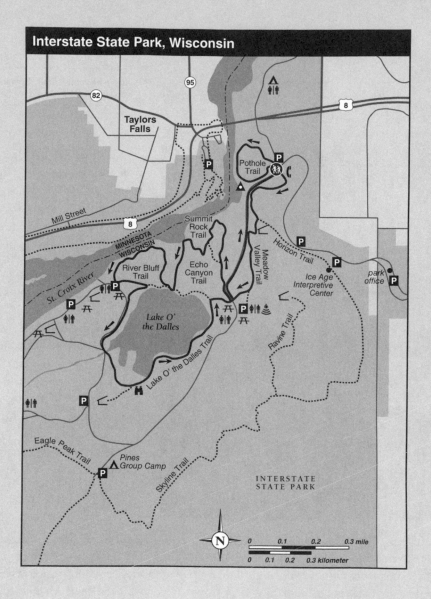

hikes that ultimately combine to form a winding trail through huge boulder fields, lava flows, and glacial features. Leave your car behind, and follow the trail west as it snakes through huge boulders and around scattered pine trees and stunted oaks on its way to the bluffs above the river. The trail inches along to the edge of the bluff, about 50 feet to the river below, then turns to the right over a wooden footbridge. The footbridge leads the hiker over not a chasm in the rocks, but one of the large potholes cut into the hard, rocky bluff.

About 1 billion years ago, this very spot was being covered in lava oozing out of the ground about 100 miles north of the Dalles of the St. Croix. Thousands of cubic miles of lava spread across this area. The colossal weight of the lava sagged

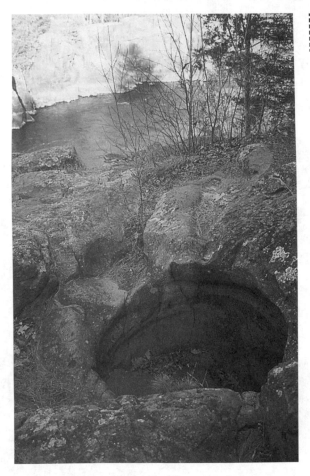

Along the Pothole Trail, the work of volcanoes and glaciers is evident.

in the middle, making a gigantic basin—and that basin eventually filled with water. Today we call that expanse of water Lake Superior.

Later pre-Cambrian and Cambrian layers of sand and gravel from ancient seas were deposited over this lava. Between then and about 1 million years ago, countless rivers and streams cut through the sandstone, exposing the lava below. Erosion over eons scraped and smoothed the lava, sometimes cutting channels through it.

About 1 million years ago, the first of many ice ages advanced on the area, which further contributed to the sculpting of the landscape. One result of the ice age is the many circular pits or holes seemingly bored into the lava. These potholes were formed when a boulder or rock got caught in a depression or crack in the lava. Unable to be washed away, a boulder would continue to tumble around and around in these depressions. Sand and smaller rocks would get washed into the holes as they were continually scoured deeper and deeper by the grinding boulder. Some of the resulting potholes are more than 60 feet deep and nearly 10 feet in diameter. Many smaller ones can be found scattered throughout the rocks here and across the river in Minnesota.

Leave the potholes, and continue along the top of the bluff as you admire spectacular views of the river. Rock climbers enjoy these bluffs, and the trail passes a popular rappelling spot on the nearby bluff top. Shortly after the trail swings to the right, there is an observation platform offering a grand view down and across the river.

The trail intersects several spurs—all leading to points along the edge of the bluff. The designated trail climbs up to a knob that overlooks the park road to the right. At this point it swings back down and to the left and returns to the pot-hole trailhead.

Back at the parking lot, cross the park road to reach the trailhead for Horizon Rock Trail. The map shows it as a 0.5-mile linear trail, but don't worry—you're only taking it halfway as a short but rewarding side trip. Head into the woods along a creek bed and through an overstory of maple. At about 0.2 mile, you will come to a path to the right. Don't take it yet; continue straight up the slope to the top, another 0.1 mile. Here you will come to steps in the rocks and a large rock knob. Follow the trail up around the knob to the left, and you will encounter a stone shelter. The top of the knob yields a grand view of the surrounding St. Croix River valley to the south and a bird's-eye view of the town of Taylors Falls to the north. It's a quick and easy side trip.

Descend back to the trail intersection, and turn left onto the Meadow Valley Trail. Take this trail for 0.4 mile until you come to a park road at the parking lot for the amphitheater. Take the road to the right out to the main park road, and turn right again. Across the road on the left (about 150 yards) is the parking lot for two trailheads: the Summit Rock Trail and a trail to a beach house at Lake O' the Dalles. This hike continues along the Summit Rock Trail at the north end of the parking area.

The trail winds through ironwoods as it meanders its way to the bluff line. At about 0.1 mile, the trail intersects the Echo Canyon Trail on the left. Continue straight on the Summit Rock Trail through a section that winds through large boulders as it climbs toward an observation deck on the bluff. The deck is a few yards off to the right on a trail spur you take immediately before climbing up onto the bluff's edge. From that deck, you can see the river and the riverboats that carry tourists up and down the Dalles.

After visiting the observation deck, take the steps up and over the lip and then go back down more steps to a second observation deck. The trail follows along and through more boulder fields as it climbs along the bluff line. The trail tops a knoll dotted with short, gnarly oak trees. The path to the left is not the designated trail—stay to the right, and continue around the knoll.

You will soon arrive at a trail intersection on the right. This is another junction with the Echo Canyon Trail. Now you can take a right and continue on the Echo Canyon loop, yet another loop that winds through boulders and hardwood forest on the bluff top. About 0.1 mile after the T intersection, the trail cuts to the right, drops down, and becomes a bit more rough and rocky. The rock outcrops in this area reminded me of an ancient, manmade stone wall, complete with seams between the blocks of rock. The trail continues down a steep incline to the cliff edge above the river.

You will pass spurs off this section of the trail that have been closed, presumably to allow for regeneration of the trails. Echo Canyon Trail turns away from the river as you approach a large rock wall. The trail then heads up a valleylike canyon flanked by stately evergreens.

This trail comes out at the shore of Lake O' the Dalles. The T intersection offers you a chance to go left toward the bathhouse and the start of this section of the trails at the parking lot. However, to continue hiking, turn right at the T, and head back for more boulders, maple overstory, and views from the bluff.

About 100 yards down the lakeshore, the River Bluff Trail veers off to the right and up into the woods. You'll pass a small bog on your left and gain a little elevation as you ascend toward more boulder outcrops before approaching the top of the bluff again. There are more open vistas of the river as this trail circles around and drops down a moderately steep, sloping trail that comes out at the River Picnic Shelters road.

At the bottom of the trail, just as it hits the level park grounds, a small deer trail to the left will take you back to Lake O' the Dalles. Take the left, and continue along the deer path, through the understory at the edge of the woods, and you will come out at a T intersection at the lake's shoreline. Take a right, follow the lake around to its southern end, meet up with the park road to cross over the creek, and continue along the eastern shore of the lake. This is the Lake O' the Dalles Trail, part of the 1-mile loop around this 23-acre lake.

The first intersection leads back to the Camp Interstate Shelter. Stay to the left for about another 0.4 mile until you arrive at the beach house. Turn right to follow a section you passed earlier; then stop at the parking lot and intersection with the park road. Either hike 0.5 mile up the park road to get your car, or backtrack along the Meadow Valley Trail.

NEARBY ACTIVITIES

Besides other great trails in this park, remember Interstate State Park's Minnesota twin across the river, which is well worth a visit, too.

KINNICKINNIC STATE PARK, WISCONSIN 54

IN BRIEF

One of many rivers flowing into the St. Croix on the Minnesota–Wisconsin border, the Kinnickinnic River offers a hot trout-fishing stream, long sandy riverbanks, and a mix of hardwood forests and restored prairie meadows to hike through on this small piece of Wisconsin countryside.

DESCRIPTION

The Kinnickinnic River is one of many that flow down from Wisconsin's unglaciated western boundary into Minnesota's border rivers such as the Mississippi and, in this case, the St. Croix. Renowned as an active trout stream, its fast-flowing waters push sediment out into the St. Croix, where it settles to form the Kinnickinnic delta, reducing the width of that river's channel by half. It was the mouth of this river that first drew attention to the area as a prime candidate for a Wisconsin park.

Soon after the first series of Wisconsin parks was established, the mouth of the Kinni River, as the river is called, was among several chosen as future park sites. However, little was done for many decades. As the Twin Cities began to encroach upon the natural areas of eastern Minnesota, concerned landowners began a process to protect the area around the river. Parcels of land totaling 45 acres were donated to secure the prospect of

KEY AT-A-GLANCE INFORMATION

LENGTH: 3.2 miles

CONFIGURATION: Loop

DIFFICULTY: Mostly level; easy

SCENERY: Bluff tops and meadows, surprisingly few glimpses of the river

EXPOSURE: Mostly full sun; some shade

TRAFFIC: Mostly trout fishers on the river; swimmers on the beach and in delta area

TRAIL SURFACE: Mowed grass; earthen

HIKING TIME: 1–1.5 hours

SEASON: Year-round; would be good cross-country ski trail

ACCESS: $7 daily for Wisconsin residents, $10 out-of-state; $25 annual pass for Wisconsin residents, $35 out-of-state

MAPS: Available at park information kiosk at end of parking lot, or at www.dnr.state.wi.us/org/land/parks/specific/kinnickinnic

FACILITIES: Drinking water, pit toilet, picnic area, swimming beach

SPECIAL COMMENTS: Swimming in the St. Croix River is very popular here.

CONTACT: (715) 425-1129

Directions

From south St. Paul, go south on US 10/61 to Prescott, Wisconsin. Take WI 35 North (left) up the hill, and then turn left (north) on CR F for about 5 miles to 820th Avenue. Turn left, and drive 0.2 mile to park entrance on left. Follow road all the way to end by picnic area.

GPS TRAILHEAD COORDINATES

Latitude   N92° 45.690'

Longitude   W44° 49.807'

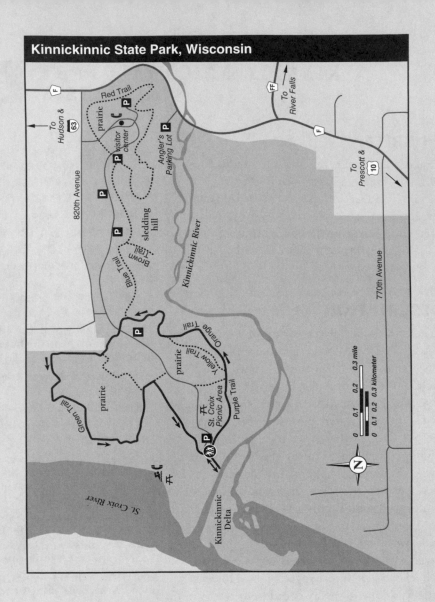

Kinnickinnic State Park, Wisconsin

a Kinnickinnic State Park. The Wisconsin Department of Natural Resources was impressed by this show of support, and the park was established in 1972.

Since then, more than 20,000 trees have been planted by volunteers, and more than 50 acres of prairie have been restored. Bird-watchers should note that more than half of the birds listed for Wisconsin have been found in this park—and more during migration. Even in winter this is a good place to spot birds; because of the flow of the water from the Kinni into the St. Croix, the river around the delta doesn't freeze, making it a natural gathering area for bald eagles during the cold months. More than 140 species of birds have been identified in the park, and it's estimated that upwards of 90 species could be seen at any one time during spring migration. This represents about 50% of Wisconsin's nesting bird species. Wild turkeys were reintroduced into the park in 1989—though this locale is approaching the northern limit of their natural range.

This hike consists of a series of connecting trails forming a loop that showcases those uplands and bluffs that give this river its character. Each trail is marked with colored, banded posts that correspond to the color guide on the trail map.

The hike begins at the west end of the parking lot, following a paved path past the picnic areas to an impressive overlook above the Kinnickinnic River, right where it spills into the St. Croix below. Retrace your steps to the Purple Trail, which leads off to the right as you are coming back from the overlook. Follow the top of the bluff line beside the picnic area before heading into the woods. These woods are typical of upper bluff forests in this part of Wisconsin: oaks and maples with some ashes mixed in. The understory is dense and lush as the trail meanders through a narrow corridor framed by branches and foliage.

At about 0.4 mile, the trail intersects with the Orange Trail. Take the right fork, and continue along the wooded bluffs high above the river. Below are the swift, clear-running, trout-filled waters of the Kinni River, popular with fly fishermen who like the wide stretches as it runs through the park. The trout is the exceptionally large German brown trout. The Kinni is a Category V trout stream, which means there are certain restrictions and daily bag limits. You must also have a valid Wisconsin or out-of-state fishing license to fish this river.

The Orange Trail wanders for about 0.2 mile before it intersects with the Yellow Trail. Stay to the right, and continue on the Orange. You are skirting one of the restored prairies of the park at this point. Continue another 0.4 mile to the intersection with the Blue Trail, which leads east toward a series of trails around the park entrance. Save those for a side trip and instead take the left fork, which is now considered the Yellow Trail. This will cross the park road just to the east (right) of a parking lot at the prairie area.

This hike continues into the prairie meadows for about another 0.1 mile until you intersect with the Green Trail. Turn right to follow this 1.4-mile trail that loops around the northern section of the park, skirting the prairie and more of the upland woods common here. It rejoins with the Yellow Trail about 0.1 mile before that trail crosses the park road. However, at about 100 yards beyond the intersection with the Yellow Trail (just before the road), there is a trail off to the right, the northern end of the Purple Trail. The Purple Trail parallels the park road and hugs the bluff above the swimming area before joining up with the picnic grounds where this hike started.

NEARBY ACTIVITIES

Try some trout fishing in the Kinnickinnic River, or take a scenic drive along the Wisconsin bank of the St. Croix, either north to Hudson or south to Prescott.

55   PINE POINT REGIONAL PARK TRAIL

KEY AT-A-GLANCE INFORMATION

LENGTH: 3.6 miles

CONFIGURATION: Three interconnected loops

DIFFICULTY: Easy overall; some hills, and some soft and muddy sections; trails seem longer than on map.

SCENERY: Mostly upland forests with one big meadow and a few lakes a short distance off trail

EXPOSURE: Mixed full sun with dense shade

TRAFFIC: Bicyclists on Munger Trail; hiking trails more secluded

HIKING TIME: 2–3 hours

TRAIL SURFACE: Packed earth or mowed turf; wet in boggy areas

SEASON: Year-round; some segments part of cross-country network

ACCESS: No fees at Pine Point; other Washington County Parks: $5 daily vehicle permit, $25 annual permit; Washington County, Anoka, and Carver County Park each honor the other counties' passes

MAPS: At bulletin board in park and www.co.washington.mn.us/parks

FACILITIES: Restrooms, drinking water, picnic tables

SPECIAL COMMENTS: Some trails are shared with horses. Be prepared for lots of biting insects in July.

CONTACT: (651) 430-8370

GPS TRAILHEAD COORDINATES

Latitude   N92° 50.277'

Longitude   W45° 7.240'

IN BRIEF

Pine Point Regional Park has a robust hiking trail and is a major trailhead for the Willard Munger State Trail, which serves as the backbone of this park.

DESCRIPTION

Pine Point Regional Park sits close to the eastern end of the Willard Munger State Trail, whose eastern terminus is only a few miles beyond this park. While much of the park's trail use occurs on this wide, paved expressway for bikers, skaters, and hikers, it's the other network of walking trails that really introduces hikers to this park's character. Also, keep in mind that the trails at Pine Point, except for the paved one, are shared with horseback riders.

This hike follows an irregular, amoeba-shaped trail through Pine Point Regional Park and captures virtually every area and amenity the park has to offer. Start right behind the information bulletin board to the right of the restrooms at the end of the parking lot. The state trail leads right behind the bulletin board, but cross it and angle to the left. A few feet farther you'll see a 6-foot-wide grassy pathway into the woods. Look for a signpost (Intersection 5) marking the trailhead.

The trail is sandy and winds through oaks and spruces and a split stand of white pines on

----

Directions ⟶

From St. Paul, drive north on I-694 to MN 36 toward Stillwater. Take CR 5 north through Stillwater to the intersection with SR 96. CR 5 becomes CR 55. Take CR 55 north about 3 miles to park entrance on left. Park at far end of lot near restrooms.

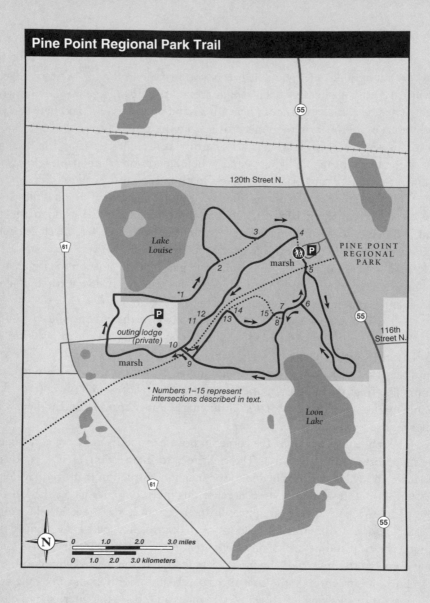

Pine Point Regional Park Trail

Lake Louise

marsh

PINE POINT REGIONAL PARK

*1

2

3

4

5

6

7

8

11 12 13 14 15

10

9

outing lodge
(private)

marsh

Loon Lake

120th Street N.

116th Street N.

55

61

61

55

55

* Numbers 1–15 represent
intersections described in text.

N

0   1.0   2.0   3.0 miles

0   1.0   2.0   3.0 kilometers

the right, red pines on the left. A note of warning: I hiked this trail one early morning during midsummer and experienced hundreds of mosquitoes and deer flies.

The trail bends to the left through a stand of red pines before swinging back around through a low area near the park's boundary. This lobe is about 0.3 mile out and another 0.3 mile back to the next intersection. At the end of the lobe, the trail crosses a low-lying area that can be muddy after lots of rain. Birch, box elder, aspen, and spruce trees line the trail as you climb back up toward Intersection 6.

At Intersection 6, where the trail intersects at a T, take the left trail toward Intersection 7 on the map. You will come to Intersection 7 about 50 yards down the trail. Keep to the left, and go another 50 yards past Intersection 8. You are now on a long, 0.4-mile lobe that brings you first along the top western edge of Loon Lake on your left and then swings around to skirt a large meadow on your right. There is a thick understory beneath a stand of aspens and oaks between you and the lake, so you won't see much of it from the trail.

This section of the trail gets very narrow as it climbs up from the lake and out of the trees through a lighter stand of box elders and white maples. It has the character of a deer trail or a worn hikers' path in the north woods.

This trail intersects with the Munger Trail at Intersection 9. Take the paved trail to the left for about 10 yards, and then make a right into the woods across the trail to Intersection 10. If you imagine this entire route as a big, albeit irregular, figure eight, you are now at the center of the figure eight, between the loops.

Follow the (muddy) trail to the left, and pass a boggy area on the right. After a sharp right at a small pond (on your left), the trail now leads north and across a segment that actually lies outside the official park boundary.

You will come to a paved road that leads into the private Outing Lodge area to your right. Cross the road, and continue on the trail cut into the thicket on the other side. There's no sign, but it's very clear this is the trail. The trail continues as a narrow pathway through mixed buckthorns, box elders, and red pines. The trees thin out a bit, and as you pass a row of scotch pines (they have orange bark toward the top of a slightly gnarly upper trunk) you can barely see Lake Louise in the distance.

The trail comes out along the corner of private property and then, according to the map, forks at Intersection 1. The right fork to Intersection 11 was impossible to locate on my hike, probably due to some light construction that may have obliterated the trail. It doesn't matter, because this hike continues along the left fork toward Intersection 2. As you approach Intersection 2, you'll see a field straight ahead. The trail to Intersection 3 loops to the north, first past Lake Louise, then around the cropland before joining back up at Intersection 3. It's about a 0.3-mile loop if you go to the left, or about a 0.15-mile loop if you cut straight ahead.

From Intersection 3, the trail turns south and is only about 0.1 mile from your start at the parking lot. To gain extra miles and to see the interior of the park along the Munger Trail, turn right at Intersection 4 and head back into the thicker part of the woods. The trail cuts along the edge of a wet marshy area. Scores of frogs leaped across the trail here just in front of my feet.

This narrow "deer trail" continues through a tall stand of oaks. After the pond, the trail sideswipes a gravel path that parallels the Munger Trail. This gravel trail must be relatively new since it does not appear on the park map. Don't pay any attention to it as the narrow trail is more scenic and less crowded.

This trail meets the Munger at Intersection 12, but stay on the trail until you come to the signpost for Intersection 11. This trail, if followed to the right, takes you back to the corner of the private property at Intersection 1. Stay on your narrow path, past Intersection 11, and go another 0.1 mile to Intersection 10. You have just completed the upper loop of the figure eight and are back at the middle. From this point you technically backtrack along a trail that returns to the trailhead.

Take a left at Intersection 10, and cross the Munger Trail again, this time heading toward the meadow at Intersection 9. Turn left toward Intersection 13 about 0.2 mile farther. This segment follows along the southern side of the Munger Trail, passes Intersection 13 on the left, and continues on to Intersection 14, where it forks. Take either fork as they both end up at Intersection 15. From Intersection 15, you'll head to Intersection 7, which is a left turn if you've come from the left fork but lies straight ahead if you came up the right fork. Either way, you want to go toward Intersection 7, where you will retrace a short, 100-yard segment of the trail you hiked much earlier (the section between Intersections 6 and 7). Now you are hiking it in reverse to reach Intersection 6 again, where you take a left back up to the trailhead at Intersection 5, and the parking lot.

NEARBY ACTIVITIES

Stillwater to the south is full of shops. The quaint river village of Marine on St. Croix and William O'Brien State Park (see page 249) are a few minutes' drive north.

56 RED CEDAR STATE TRAIL, WISCONSIN

KEY AT-A-GLANCE INFORMATION

LENGTH: 14.5 miles

CONFIGURATION: Out-and-back

DIFFICULTY: Easy; flat with very few rises or dips

SCENERY: Trail runs right along the river's edge

EXPOSURE: Mostly full sun; some shade

TRAFFIC: Bicyclists along the entire route; hikers vary by segment; popular trail during summer

TRAIL SURFACE: Entire path is hard-packed crushed rock

HIKING TIME: 4.5–6 hours

SEASON: Year-round; ski trail in winter

ACCESS: No fee for hiking

MAPS: Available at trailhead visitor center (old depot), or at www.dnr .wi.gov/org/land/parks/specific /redcedar

FACILITIES: Restrooms, drinking water, picnic tables at visitor center

SPECIAL COMMENTS: Watch for bicyclists. Shuttling a car is a good idea, and you'll find parking lots at each segment intersection.

CONTACT: (715) 232-1242

GPS TRAILHEAD COORDINATES

Latitude   N91° 56.376'

Longitude   W44° 52.517'

IN BRIEF

Even though it's a state trail/biking-and-hiking corridor, it's also one of only a few trails within 60 miles of the Twin Cities to the east and across the border into Wisconsin. Also, and more important, its course along the Red Cedar River makes it an especially enjoyable route to hike—replete with history, grand vistas of the river, and great scenery.

DESCRIPTION

This is one of a few state trails that are detailed in this book. While all state trail/regional corridors in Minnesota and Wisconsin offer many more miles of hiking and biking opportunities, those in the Twin Cities area either run along busier highways, cut through backyards, or are part of former railroad rights-of-way. These are wonderful pathways in their own right. However, I think this one deserves special mention because of its remoteness and beauty.

As most rails-to-trails paths, this trail was constructed on a railroad right-of-way—in particular, a section of the Red Cedar Junction Line that served the Knapp, Stout and Company. At that time, this was the largest lumber-producing company in the world. Beginning

----

Directions ⟶

From the Twin Cities, head east into Wisconsin on I-94 and turn right (south) onto WI 25 and drive to Menomonie. To reach the trailhead, turn right (west) onto WI 29 and go across the river; take your first left and park. To leave a shuttle car at the southern end, continue south on WI 25, through Downsville, to CR Y. Take a left on CR Y, and reach the parking lot on the right, just after crossing the bridge.

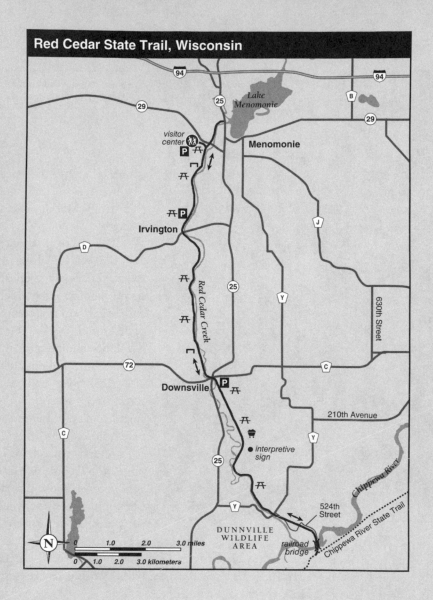

Red Cedar State Trail, Wisconsin

in the 1870s, the line operated for nearly 100 years before being abandoned in 1973, when it was acquired by the Wisconsin Department of Natural Resources for trail development. The visitor center is housed in the old railroad depot, and fortunately this 14-mile course of the railroad followed right along the banks of the Red Cedar River.

The hike begins at the end of the small park adjacent to the Red Cedar Trail Visitor Center. A brief orientation of the trail's layout and history gives hikers an introductory perspective on the 14-mile trail. From the visitor center, head to the end of the parking lot, through Riverside Park on the visitor center grounds, and on to the trailhead. Each section of the trail is labeled according to the towns it

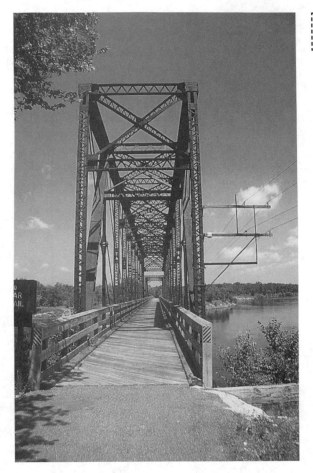

A converted railroad bridge along the Red Cedar Trail

connects along the river. The first section, 2.7 miles, runs from Menomonie to Irvington.

This is river country, and the woods along the river's edge are typically silver maples, box elders, and their representative understories of sumacs, hazelnuts, and myriad other vegetation. Higher points along the river encourage oaks and other, hardier sugar and red maples to take hold.

After roughly 1.1 miles, you'll come to a large rock face on the right, rippling with a constant sheen of water along its entire face. In the summer, these "weeping rocks" promote a healthy covering of ferns that cling to the walls. The area is actually called the Ice Palisades because in the winter, this water freezes to form a wintry shroud of ice over the entire cliff face.

Geologically speaking, the Red Cedar River is in that area of Wisconsin known as the Driftless area, where the glaciers from the most recent ice age failed to cover the land. Its terrain is therefore more rolling and otherwise different from the scoured and scored landscapes to the north.

Some maps talk of a Devil's Punch Bowl formation a bit farther down from the Palisades—on the right side just before you come into Irvington. I could not find the site. Perhaps poking more thoroughly through the thick undergrowth along this section would reveal it to bushwhackers.

The next section is 4.3 miles long and continues toward Downsville. The countryside changes a little bit through this section as it opens up more into farm country and marshes. About 1.5 miles down this section is a creek that meets the river. This is an area where archaeological digs have uncovered 3,000-year-old arrowheads. Ironically, the name Red Cedar isn't native in origin at all, but rather comes from the discovery of one red cedar tree floating in the river when French traders were exploring this area.

At Downsville the trail crosses the river and heads down its eastern bank. This section is called the Dunnville section and adds another 4.2 miles to the trail's length. The trail isn't as close to the river as it has been. This section is noted for the number of quarry sites found about halfway along. An interpretive site at mile 10 marks the location of the Dunnville Sandstone Quarry.

A mile farther, and you'll come to a bend in the river and a picnic site. Petroglyphs were once near this site but have long since been destroyed. They still may appear in some references and on some maps.

At Dunnville, you cross CR Y and enter the Dunnville Wildlife Area. A parking lot across the bridge (take a right at CR Y) can serve as the southern terminus of this trail since it's a good place to park a car if you are making this a one-way hike with a car shuttle. The trail does continue for another 2.5 miles to a long railroad bridge over the river. Just upstream from this bridge is the confluence of the Red Cedar with the Chippewa River, a moderate tributary to the Mississippi River from Wisconsin.

It's worth the walk to see this old, narrow bridge that looms across the river. An expansive sandy beach down the trail to the right, accessible just before you approach the bridge, furnishes a popular resting place for hikers and bikers. You'll even see waders and swimmers cooling off at this wide, gentle bend in the river.

From the railroad bridge, the trail continues another 26 miles as the Chippewa River State Trail. When the Red Cedar portion ends, you must backtrack to either the parking lot at CR Y, or all the way back to Menomonie. There is also designated parking at Irvington for dropping a car there along the trail.

NEARBY ACTIVITIES

Check your road map—on the way back to Minnesota you have a few options for enjoying other trails in Wisconsin's parks, including the trails within Kinnickinnic State Park (see page 231).

57 TAMARACK NATURE CENTER

KEY AT-A-GLANCE INFORMATION

LENGTH: 1.3 miles (up to 6.4 miles of trails available)

CONFIGURATION: Full circle loop from visitor center with many optional routes

DIFFICULTY: Easy; mostly level

SCENERY: Lots of birches and aspens surrounded by grasslands and alder marshes

EXPOSURE: Mostly full sun; some shade

TRAFFIC: Stay in center of park to avoid ambient highway noise; trails busier nearer the nature center

TRAIL SURFACE: Paved trails, earthen paths, and wooden walkways

HIKING TIME: 45–60 minutes

SEASON: Year-round; skiing and snowshoeing popular in winter

ACCESS: No fees

MAPS: Available at visitor center or www.co.ramsey.mn.us/parks/tamarack

FACILITIES: Nature center, restrooms, drinking water; ample parking in lot at visitor center entrance

SPECIAL COMMENTS: A haven for wildlife, this park also offers informative signage for the indigenous trees along an interpretive route.

CONTACT: (651) 407-5350

GPS TRAILHEAD COORDINATES

Latitude   N93° 2.335'

Longitude   W45° 6.066'

IN BRIEF

This 1-square-mile patch of nature offers a short, easy hike through a marsh setting, typical of many of the forested regions of central Minnesota. The Play Area and Discovery Garden are now open.

DESCRIPTION

For a compact natural area surrounded by freeways, Tamarack Nature Center offers a pleasant example of north woods diversity. The only thing missing at the Tamarack Nature Center—tamarack trees! Wildlife abounds and the setting takes you to the marshy alder bogs of northern Minnesota. While there are several alternate routes within this small park, this hike passes through the heart of the park and is probably the quietest path.

Immediately behind the visitor center, you'll see an 8-acre prairie-restoration project. Prairie grasses and wildflowers dominate this otherwise open, flat field characteristic of the prairie meadows that once dominated this region.

The 5-foot-wide paved pathway here is great for either wheelchairs or strollers, and it basically makes a loop around the restoration project. You'll also begin the hike here. When ready, head right (north) along the Prairie Trail.

Directions ⟶

This center is unmarked on many maps. Take I-35 East north from St. Paul to CR H-2 (about 1.7 miles north of MN 96). Exit eastward (right) to Otter Lake Road (CR 60). Turn south (right), and drive to park entrance (about 300 yards). Trailhead starts at far end of lot near interpretive center.

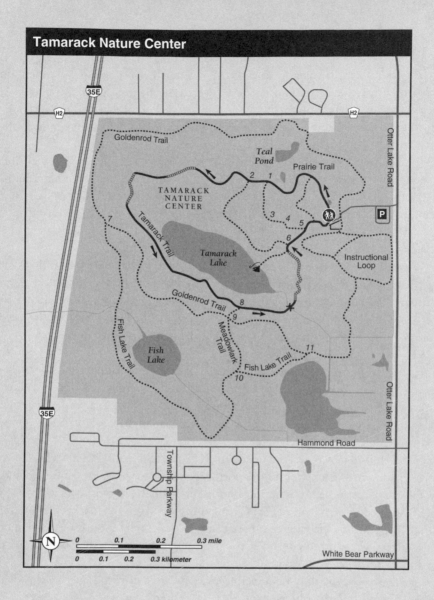

Goldenrod Trail

Teal
Pond

Prairie Trail

2 1

TAMARACK
NATURE
CENTER

3   4
5

7

Tamarack Trail

6

P

Instructional
Loop

Tamarack
Lake

Goldenrod Trail   8

9

Meadowlark Trail

11

Fish Lake Trail

Fish Lake Trail

Fish
Lake

10

Hammond Road

Township Parkway

N

| 0 | 0.1 | 0.2 | 0.3 mile |
| 0 | 0.1 | 0.2 | 0.3 kilometer |

White Bear Parkway

Otter Lake Road

35E

H2

H2

35E

About 700 feet down the trail, you'll come to a small wooded area of aspens and oaks surrounding a smaller pond. This is Teal Pond, and it offers a modest observation deck at the end of a very short spur trail. About 200 feet past that turnout is Intersection 1, clearly marked on the left. The paved path sweeps left, but you want to make a right at the Intersection 1 marker and continue around the east side of Tamarack Lake. You'll come upon Intersection 2 a short distance farther. This, too, goes through the wooded area bordering the restoration area but keeps more toward the marshy edges of Tamarack Lake. Again, stay to the right for a longer hike.

Now called the Tamarack Trail, this path continues through another small stand of woods and then back through more open grasses and islands of trees. It circles around another marshy area to the north before becoming a wooden footpath along the edge of yet another marshy area on the left. There are quite a few deer in this area (based on the many deer tracks). Those tracks and my sighting of four deer just beyond the wooden walkway in the middle of the day indicate that the deer are plentiful and not too shy with hikers.

At the northwest end of the park, the trail cuts south through a thick stand of alders and marsh grass. The alders are quite tall in this area, creating a tunnel-like walk beneath their canopy. Once you've crossed this neck of marsh, you are facing a long, grass-covered hill that appears to be the highest elevation in the park. The trail turns to the left and passes beside the tree line growing along the edge of Tamarack Lake and the grass cover on the right.

About 0.4 mile after you come out of the alders, you'll hit Intersection 8 and the Meadowlark Trail, which opens up a number of hike alternatives as it goes southward and disappears over the ridge. Taking this trail will connect hikers with Fish Lake Trail and channel them either east about 0.7 mile back to the visitor center or out to the trails that follow along the park's western perimeter.

However, our hike continues along the edge of the lake for another 600 feet before reentering the alder-thicketed marsh area at the southern end of the lake. There is a small footbridge followed by an extensive section of wooden walkway. Both ends of the lake are good birding areas. This marshy area, while not totally appealing as a scenic feature, nevertheless is representative of such vast marshy areas in Minnesota and elsewhere.

The trail comes out at Intersection 6. Turn right onto the stretch of paved trail, which circles back around the northern route to the visitor center. This and later sections form part of the interpretive loop that offers information on the trees you encounter en route. Head straight until you see the marker for Intersection 5 (the trails to the right are part of the instructional loop for cross-country skiers in the winter), and continue straight, back toward the visitor center and the origin of your hike.

Interestingly, the only tamarack trees I saw were growing outside the visitor center. There is a large one just south of the center's back side, right next to the trail, and another alongside the building. (For a great opportunity to walk among the tamaracks, check out the hike listing for Tamarack Trail, page 171.)

NEARBY ACTIVITIES

This park is only about 15 minutes north of Vadnais–Snail Lake if you want to put more hiking adventures on your plate.

WILD RIVER STATE PARK 58

IN BRIEF

One of several state parks along the upper St. Croix River, Wild River offers a pleasant walk along the river's banks. Forests regenerated after decades of lumber harvesting are now mature stands of oaks and maples. Together the river and forest offer many of the natural amenities for which Minnesota parks are renowned.

DESCRIPTION

Always a great river to paddle, the St. Croix is equally rewarding from a hiker's perspective— St. Croix Wild River State Park presents a scenic river walk coupled with a hike through dense stands of Minnesota hardwoods.

This hike begins at the edge of the river, near the canoe-rental site. At the turnaround, head south along the trail, which is marked several ways: Amik's Pond loop, River Trail, and Deer Creek. All follow the same path from the trailhead sign at the edge of the road.

The trail is a 6-foot-wide mowed, earthen path that follows the river a little more than 0.2 mile before turning inland and upland. At 0.2 mile, the Amik's Pond loop turnoff leads off to the right. Stay to the left along the river for a few more yards before the main trail turns to the right. You will leave the cover of ashes

----

Directions

From Minneapolis, take I-35 West north to MN 95 in North Branch (Exit 147). Take MN 95 right (east) about 10 miles to CR 12 in Almelund. Turn left (north), and go 3 miles to park entrance. Drive into park, take second major right, and follow sign to canoe-rental/launch area. Park in the lot to the left of the canoe-rental shed.

KEY AT-A-GLANCE INFORMATION

LENGTH: 4.6 miles

CONFIGURATION: Loop

DIFFICULTY: Easy; level, only a few inclines; some sandy areas by river

SCENERY: The St. Croix valley at its finest; river stays in view for about half this hike

EXPOSURE: Full shade except for meadow crossings

TRAFFIC: Little along the river; campground and picnic areas utilized on weekends; boat ramps popular

TRAIL SURFACE: About 40% paved trail; 60% earthen or mowed grass with some sandy areas

HIKING TIME: 2–2.5 hours

SEASON: Year-round; winter ski trails

ACCESS: Minnesota State Park fee system: $5 daily, $25 annual permit, $12 annual permit for disabled individuals

MAPS: Available at park headquarters or at www.dnr.state.mn.us /state_parks/wild_river

FACILITIES: Campground, picnic area, restrooms, showers, drinking water, canoe rental, boat launch

SPECIAL COMMENTS: Expect to see lots of canoes on the river. The park is a good place to stop for a hike while canoeing.

CONTACT: (651) 583-2125

GPS TRAILHEAD COORDINATES

Latitude   N92° 43.769'

Longitude   W45° 31.366'

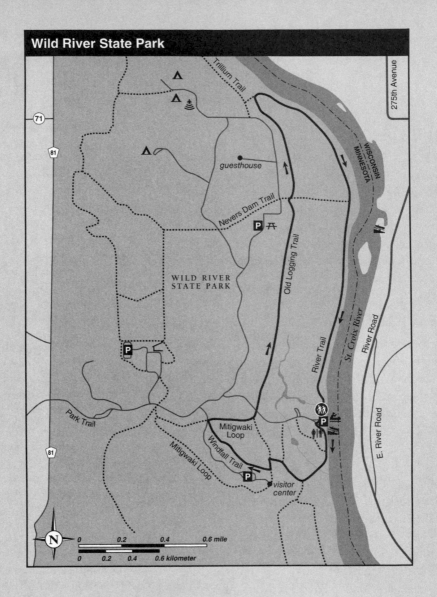

and willows and head toward a stand of birches at the back edge of a meadow (check for deer in the early morning). You will then come to a T in the trail. The left branch of the T turns south and becomes the Deer Creek Trail—also a horse trail. Stay to the right, and continue around the southern end of Amik's Pond. This area, like the rest of the park, is alive with birds. Expect to see eastern pewees, mourning doves, Baltimore orioles, and warblers along the trail. For the next 0.2 mile you should also notice signage and interpretive points along this portion of the Amik's Pond interpretive trail.

At the next intersection, the Amik's Pond Trail spur goes right; stay left to follow the Windfall Trail, another interpretive trail. You'll come upon a sign leading you to the Old Logging Trail and then the Old Logging Trail itself. The trail climbs a bit, past a thick understory of ferns and ashes and oak saplings.

At the intersection of this wide, paved trail, hang a left and go about 100 yards to the remaining section of the Windfall Trail. Take this trail to the right to continue the loop. You will pass through a mature stand of oaks, ashes, and birches—a stately forest of older trees and a grand sampling of some of Minnesota's noble hardwoods.

About halfway along this section, you'll come to a turnout on your left with a bench and a strange wood, tablelike contraption. This is a tree-finder and identifier, and it's pretty easy to figure out. Windows contain descriptions and illustrations of some of the major tree species in the area (ironwood, basswood, oak, and so on). Once you center the information in the window, two sights line up that allow you to find that tree in the cluster growing around the tree finder. Look through the eyehole; check out the tree that aligns with the V notch in the other end and you've located the tree highlighted in the information window.

When you come to a signpost marked 4, you have intersected the Mitigwaki Trail, a paved trail that you want to take to the right for 0.2 mile to rejoin the Old Logging Trail. You'll come to a T, at which point you'll take a left to head north. You'll soon cross a park road, but keep going straight, into the heart of the forest.

Up to now you've sampled the southern half of the park's hiking trails—to the south and west, horse trails prevail. However, the Old Logging Trail is a wide avenue through a mature stand of upland hardwoods. For the next mile you'll experience a peaceful walk through the upland woods of near-northern Minnesota.

While hiking along this section, imagine loggers felling trees, trimming them, and loading trunks onto large wagons that drove up and down such roads. Much of the logging was done in winter, when roads were solid and underbrush was at a minimum. In this significant logging region, many roads like this one served as major arteries for getting the lumber to the rivers for the float south to sawmills on the St. Croix River.

After a mile, the trail opens onto the developed picnic area. Several facilities are available here, including drinking water, restrooms, a pavilion, and barbecue pits. At the far end of the pavilion, turn right (east) onto the Nevers Dam Trail. Almost immediately there is a cut to the left. This is the River Terrace Loop, a 1-mile trail that meets up with the St. Croix at 0.5 mile and then swings south (to the right) along the river and back to the Nevers Dam site. Unless you want to cut off 1 mile of hiking to get to the Nevers Dam site (only 0.2 mile to the river), take the River Terrace Loop to the left.

At the top of the River Terrace Loop is a trail to the left called the Trillium Trail. This trail heads northwest toward the northern corner of the park where it meets up with the Sunrise Trail and actually continues upstream along the St. Croix to another park unit section on the Sunrise River. There's also a long staircase that leads to the campground. Save this hike for another day, and continue around the loop to the right and back toward the river.

The trail follows the river for 0.5 mile before coming to the Nevers Dam site. There, an interpretive sign will tell you about this dam, which was built to hold back logs awaiting processing at the lumber mills downstream at Stillwater. This dam, built in 1889, was in operation until 1954. Before the dam was built, huge logjams plugged the river for weeks, costing lumber companies a lot of money in time and damaged or destroyed logs. In 1886, a massive logjam—containing enough timber to build 15,000 houses—blocked the river in this section for more than six weeks. More than 100 logging camps used the St. Croix to move their timber south.

From the observation deck at the dam site, the trail spur heads back toward the picnic area. You want to take the trail leading off to the left as you face uphill and away from the river. This continues your river hike, and the trail now becomes the River Trail.

The trail follows the lowlands of the St. Croix, sometimes crossing sandbars that turn the trail into a brush-covered beach in spots. It stays close to the river for all of its 1.2-mile length back to the turnaround at the canoe-rental site. About halfway along the trail, a bench is conveniently placed atop the bank. It's a pleasant place to rest and enjoy the slow-flowing St. Croix.

At about 0.9 mile, you will reach a canoe campsite directly off the trail to the right. After 20 yards, another trail enters the woods on the right. This is a walk-in backpackers' campsite accessible from the canoe-rental parking lot. It's a spacious, shaded campsite with a picnic table, a fire ring, a primitive latrine, and wonderfully flat and smooth tent spaces. If you want a great way to enjoy this hike, come in the night before, camp here, and start out on the trail bright and early the next morning. You are only 0.3 mile from the start of the trail at this point.

From the campsites, the trail veers away from the river to go around a slough on the left. It then crosses over the slough via a footbridge and comes out onto a lane about 100 yards from the canoe-rental complex (which has a road turnaround, parking lot, restroom, picnic table, and boat access to the river). At the canoe-rental shed, take a right back to the parking lot to complete this hike.

NEARBY ACTIVITIES

The northern section of the park includes the Sunrise River, another popular canoeing route. Not too much farther south is William O'Brien State Park.

WILLIAM O'BRIEN STATE PARK,
Upper Park Trail

IN BRIEF

Besides its natural beauty and the St. Croix River, the big appeal of William O'Brien State Park is its proximity to the Twin Cities. A nice hiking loop follows the river's edge in the lower park complex, but a hiker really gets a workout exploring all the loops and side trails in the network of the upper park.

DESCRIPTION

This hike begins at the interpretive center and is aptly named the Upper Park Trail. Geologically speaking, the St. Croix valley was cut by glaciers more than 10,000 years ago. Remnants of that action are evident beside the river, in the deep gorges cut into the sandstone and lava-deposited rock. Upland, evidence of the glaciers includes rolling hills, potholes, and boulders of various sizes strewn throughout the forests and meadows. All of these upland clues are visible along this trail.

From the center, head out behind the building to the trailhead sign. Carry a map with you as each trail intersection is numbered for easy orientation. The spur from the interpretive center intersects with a broad trail a couple of hundred yards past the center. Take a right to get onto the main loop. You will see

KEY AT-A-GLANCE INFORMATION

LENGTH: 4.6 miles

CONFIGURATION: Loop

DIFFICULTY: Easy, with gradual elevation changes

SCENERY: Uplands, away from river; large meadows with wildflowers; mature stands of hardwoods; expansive marsh area

EXPOSURE: Mostly full sun; some shade

TRAFFIC: Popular park, but most activity occurs down by the river

TRAIL SURFACE: Some mowed grass; other earthen pathway

HIKING TIME: 2–3 hours

SEASON: Year-round

ACCESS: Minnesota State Park fee system: $5 daily, $25 annual permit, $12 annual permit for disabled individuals

MAPS: At park headquarters or at www.dnr.state.mn.us/state_parks /william_obrien

FACILITIES: None in upper park beyond center's restrooms; water and campground in lower park

SPECIAL COMMENTS: This part of park is much less seen by most visitors. Wildflowers bloom in profusion during summer, particularly in meadows near the center.

CONTACT: (651) 433-0500

GPS TRAILHEAD COORDINATES

Latitude	N92° 46.103'
Longitude	W45° 13.367'

Directions

From St. Paul, take I-694 North to US 61 North. In Dellwood turn right (east) onto MN 96, and drive east for about 9 miles to the intersection at the St. Croix River with MN 95. Turn left (north), and follow the road for another 9 miles through the city of Marine on St. Croix to park entrance on left. Take park road to T intersection, turn left, and then make an immediate right into interpretive center parking lot.

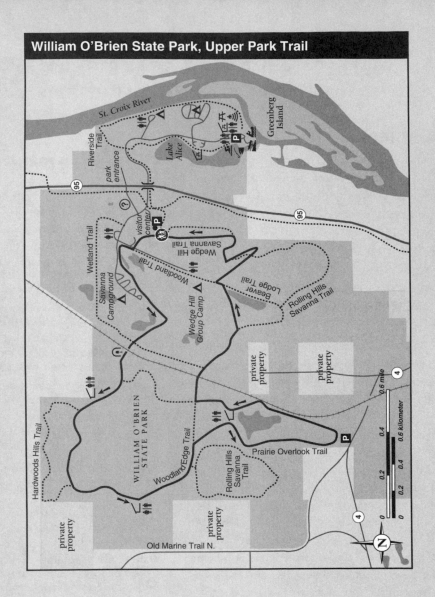

the maintenance building ahead of you, and the trail will swing to the left across a park road. This intersection with the park road is Intersection 1.

The upper park area contains a mix of hardwoods and meadows. The first part of the trail meanders through box elders and a mixed conifer forest of spruces and pines.

After you cross the road, turn right and continue behind the campgrounds; you are skirting a boglike area on the left. Its rushes indicate a moist, soggy soil. Box elder, ironwood, and basswood trees also hint at a lowland type of ecosystem common to this area. As the trail rises in elevation, white pines come into view and you will pass several trail spurs leading back to the campground on the right. This higher-elevation transition continues along the trail as you pass sumac, cedar, and oak trees.

Soon after passing the campground, be on the watch for a monstrous basswood on the right—its big, heart-shaped leaves and gigantic size will be a giveaway. These trees are also called lindens, particularly when used in landscaping. Be careful while gazing up at this giant, as the trail is flanked with a thick growth of poison ivy in this section.

Just before Intersection 2, at a sharp bend in the trail to the right, you'll come through a corridor of oaks and ironwoods. There is a bench right at the bend in the trail, and the trees in the marshy area to the right are all dead. At first, one would think the marshy area developed sometime after the trees were established and eventually drowned them out. A closer inspection of the trees' lower trunks shows clear signs of charring from a fire.

An interpretive sign later in the trail does indicate that a controlled burn took place here. Burns are used to reduce excessive understory, clean up accumulated deadfall, and encourage new growth. Some seeds need heat to break their tough seed coats, so a brush fire oftentimes is the only way they can germinate. New sprouts from regenerated plants attract wildlife into an area as well. This beneficial use of fire helps keep areas healthy.

The trail passes through this boggy area and comes to major Intersection 3 right before a foot tunnel appears under the railroad tracks. You could take either a left or a right to make this a much shorter walk or, as this hike does, continue under the tracks (follow the Hiking Club Trail sign) and head for Intersection 4 as shown on the map.

At Intersection 4 you will have hiked about 1.6 miles, and once again you have the option to alter the hike by heading south to parallel the train tracks. Otherwise, keep going straight toward Intersection 5 as this brings you into higher country. The elevation at the bog was about 840 feet. You'll climb to about 1,020 feet if you stay on this trail and continue along the main route between Intersections 5 and 8. The path crosses the face of three small ravines and skirts the northwesternmost parts of the park. About halfway along this loop, you'll come to a shelter and toilet. There is also a trail to the left that cuts back through the middle of this particular loop; it does not appear on the maps. It may be only a winter ski trail, but it can be hiked and it comes out just before Intersection 5.

After looping around the northern portion of upper woodlands and meadows, the trail comes to Intersection 8; the trail to the right leads to a firebreak loop. Stay on the main trail, and continue to Intersection 9. To shorten the hike by a mile, continue straight to Intersection 11. Otherwise head right (south) to follow a 1.5-mile loop that encompasses one of the few lakes in this section. The trail reaches its southern terminus and goes north again, eventually descending a hill into a meadow area. Just before Intersection 11, a diagonal spur to the right offers a shortcut; go ahead and take it, and turn right at the next intersection, heading east.

Go up and over the railroad tracks to Intersection 12. A word of caution: these are active tracks, but there are no warning flashers, so be sure to watch for approaching trains. Continue past Intersection 12 for 0.3 mile to Intersection 13. Along the way, you'll see a marshy area sprawled out before you. This pleasant vista gives you a sense of how the marshy areas integrate with the woods.

You will cross what appears to be a causeway, a raised trail bed across the wet, boggy area. I would expect to see an occasional water bird in this area, perhaps more so during spring and fall migration. Plenty of songbirds make their home in this park, including woodpeckers, bluebirds, orioles, herons, and a variety of warblers.

Bird-watchers may want to turn right at Intersection 13 and hike an extra 0.6-mile loop to take in the small pond just south of here. Otherwise, continue east to Intersection 17.

Two distinct ridges run north and south in this upper park. One is at the western end of the bog and is the site of the railroad bed. The other runs along the trails just to the west of the visitor center. These two ridges contain the marshy area in the middle. You can really see this defined ridgeline as you walk along the trail from Intersections 13 to 17.

Turn left at Intersection 17, and then make a right shortly thereafter. This brings you up and over this wooded ridge, at a rise in elevation of about 50 feet. You'll pass under mature stands of oaks and basswoods. The trail opens onto a meadow, another small section of trees, and yet another meadow before coming to Intersection 16. Keep to the left at this junction as you walk through a stand of maples and basswoods (lots of poison ivy again, too).

The trail intersects with an unmarked trail that goes off to the left. Don't take this unmarked trail; stay on the straight course that leads you onto the prairielike meadow before you. The interpretive center and the parking lot are ahead about 0.2 mile. The walk through this prairie is particularly enjoyable in midsummer when all the wildflowers are in bloom. If you bring a wildflower book, you could spend hours identifying all the species you see.

NEARBY ACTIVITIES

All the river activity takes place in the lower part of the park. A hiking trail along the river's edge can give you an additional 1.5 miles for the day. Interstate State Park is about 15 miles north on MN 95.

WILLOW RIVER STATE PARK 60

IN BRIEF

This trail and the surrounding park surely deserve to be called a hidden gem. The park's attractiveness as a geological and culturally rich area is surpassed only by one of the most impressive waterfalls in this part of the state. Three new campgrounds, as well as a new park office with parking for access to this trail's suggested starting point, have been added in the past few years.

DESCRIPTION

All the trails in the 3,000-plus-acre Willow River State Park are designated by name—and by color. Colored posts along the route and at intersections help orient hikers as to what route they are on or intersecting. Head down the mowed spur trail at the northern end of the parking lot to reach the trailhead.

At the T intersection, you join the Pioneer Trail (yellow). Take the trail to the right toward the Grave Sites and Willow Falls Trail (blue) as indicated by the signs at the trailhead. The Willow Falls Trail appears as a wagon path, replete with ruts and a grassy, mounded center. Aspens and oaks flank the left side of the trail, while an open meadow extends to the right.

The trail leads down into a thick understory dominated by prickly ash. Soon basswoods and oaks and an island of cedar trees

KEY AT-A-GLANCE INFORMATION

LENGTH: 4.4 miles

CONFIGURATION: Loop with one out-and-back spur

DIFFICULTY: Easy to moderate, but with steep slopes to/from river

SCENERY: Waterfall is impressive; lowlands by river and upland hardwoods pleasantly typical for region

EXPOSURE: Sections of shade and sun throughout trail's course

TRAFFIC: Any trail connecting to the waterfall trail will be popular

TRAIL SURFACE: Earthen; some parts gravel, and some parts muddy

HIKING TIME: 2–3 hours, plus time to stop at the waterfall

SEASON: Year-round; some steep trails may be impassable in winter.

ACCESS: $7 daily Wisconsin residents, $10 out-of-state; $25 annual pass for Wisconsin residents, $35 out-of-state

MAPS: Available at park headquarters or at www.dnr.wi.gov/org /land/parks/specific/willowriver

FACILITIES: Restrooms, campground, drinking water, nature center, beach, boat launch

SPECIAL COMMENTS: Plan to spend some time at the falls, and bring your camera.

CONTACT: (715) 386-5931

Directions

From the Twin Cities, take I-94 to the marked exit for Willow River State Park at Mile 4 in Wisconsin. Head north on US 12/CR U for 2 miles to CR A, and go about 1.5 miles to the park entrance.

GPS TRAILHEAD COORDINATES

Latitude   N92° 40.800'

Longitude   W45° 0.796'

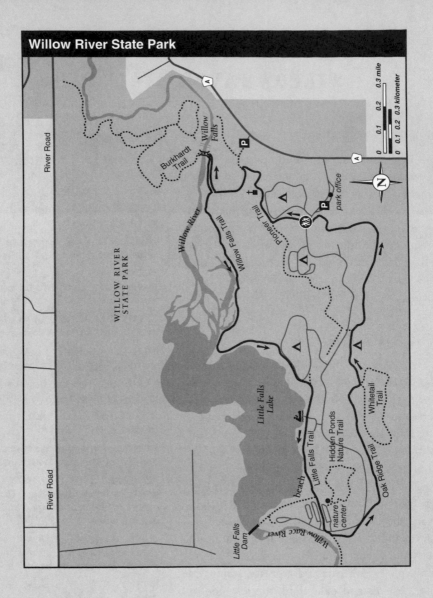

Willow River State Park

will come into view. Five hundred feet down this trail, you'll pass a small fenced section of grass that is labeled the William Scott Grave Site. The Scotts settled this area in 1849.

Although you'll find little detail about the Scotts' plight, there is much information on the history of the area in general. Prehistoric settlers in the Woodland Period practiced burying their dead in earthen mounds, many of which can still be found in the St. Croix River area nearby. Chippewa and Sioux shared this land—as enemies. Many wars broke out over the wild rice lakes in the area. One battle of record took place at the mouth of the Willow River in 1785.

Early white explorers included French, British, and American frontiersmen and traders.

The proximity to the St. Croix (the Willow River joins the St. Croix a few miles to the west at the town of Hudson, Wisconsin) made this area prime for wheat and lumber—two commodities that relied on the river for transport and commerce.

Past the gravesite, the trail continues for about 300 yards before coming to an intersection marked with a blue post. This is the trail that leads down to the river and Willow Falls. Take a left here. The right spur heads to an overlook of the falls another 300 yards farther along the bluff.

The blue trail swings steeply down into the thick of the woods, under a canopy of oaks, basswoods, and ironwoods. The trail forms a wide, deep cut into the forest floor, more like a dried creek bed than a hiking trail. It's a continuous steep drop that winds down to the river. At the riverbank you'll reach another T intersection. This is the Willow Falls Trail (blue). Ahead of you, through the trees, will be your first glimpse of a clear, trout-rich stream.

The falls are to the right, about 350 yards down the trail. Your ears will tell you what direction to go. The falls are a series of cascading steps that send up a roar of the water falling over rock down the valley. A footbridge at the base of the falls provides a continuous viewing point across the river up- and downstream. A viewing platform just before the bridge offers a great place to rest and enjoy the sounds of birds and cascading water.

The cut in the rocks through which the Willow River flows before tumbling down the rocky shelves was the site of a dam back in the wheat-producing era.

The dam was one of several built by Christian Burkhardt, a German immigrant who helped develop the area's wheat industry. Influenced by hydroelectric power plants on a visit home to Germany in the late 1800s, he built several power plants in this area. Eventually Northern States Power (NSP) purchased these power plants, and when lightning damaged one of the plants in 1963, NSP decided it was no longer profitable to maintain them. In 1967, negotiations between NSP and the Wisconsin Conservation Commission created this park. The dam that was built in the gap between the two bluffs was removed in 1992.

The best time to visit the falls (which face south) for photo opportunities is in midafternoon, when the sun swings across the valley and lights the face of the falls from the front.

Across the bridge from the falls, a trail continues up to two other overlooks and a series of looped trails on the other bluff. Our hike, however, backtracks from the falls to the T intersection at the base of the hill. This time, keep going straight along the Willow Falls Trail (blue) and continue the hike downstream.

The Willow Falls Trail measures a little more than 0.9 mile long and follows the course of the river. However, you won't see the river again until you are about halfway down the trail. Burr oaks, maples, and lots of poison ivy line both sides of the corridor through the trees. Just as the trail turns from packed earth and grass to gravel, check out the stately specimens of gigantic cottonwoods on the left.

The trail veers away from the river to go around a slough. Check it out in early morning for deer or shorebirds such as egrets and great blue herons. The

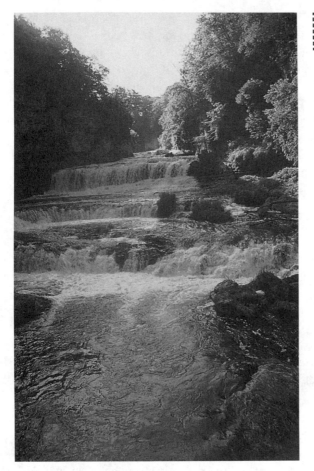

Willow River Falls

trail continues to swing left and climb as it rounds a section of the lake near the park's campgrounds. Here the Willow Falls Trail (blue) officially ends. Follow the campground roads, keeping to the right, until you come to the far end of the grounds near the campground restrooms. There you can catch the trail that heads past the boat launch and the beach. The trail is now called the Little Falls Trail (green).

Just beyond the bathhouse, the trail spurs to the right out to the dam for a nice side trip off the bigger trail loop. Back at the bathhouse, from the dam, take a right, continue about 300 yards, and cross the park road. You'll arrive at an intersection with the Trout Brook Trail (purple). Like the dam trail, this makes another short loop along the river, which adds a mile to the hike.

At the Trout Brook Trail (purple) intersection, go left along the Oak Ridge Trail (brown). This section is a mile-long stretch through some of the park's high country and stands of oaks. The Oak Ridge Trail intersects at 1 mile with the White Tail Trail (red). The Little Falls Trail (note: maps available at the park name this segment the Little Falls Trail; however, the park tabloid, also available at the park, calls this trail the Oak Ridge Trail) continues straight ahead. Or for extra mileage, you can follow the White Tail Trail to the right for a 1.2-mile loop through an open field and skirting the forest's edge. The park seems to have plenty of deer, so look for signs of their presence (such as tracks or signs of eaten bark). Stay on the Little Falls Trail/Oak Ridge Trail at this intersection by keeping to the right until you come to the park road. Immediately before crossing the road is the Knapweed Trail (orange), named for a purple-blossomed wildflower that blooms late June through mid-July. This 0.9-mile trail will take you back to the Pioneer Trail about 300 yards to the left of the parking lot where this hike started.

A shortcut at the intersection with the Knapweed Trail would be to cross the road at the orange trail and connect with the Pioneer Trail (yellow). This is about 500 yards west of the starting point at the park entrance parking lot. Take the Pioneer Trail to the right and behind the parking lot. A short spur (the same one you took from the lot at the very beginning) leads back toward the right and into the parking lot.

NEARBY ACTIVITIES

The Wisconsin community of Hudson offers small river-town charm, along with a variety of shops and restaurants.

APPENDIX
INFORMATION SOURCES

ANOKA COUNTY PARKS AND RECREATION
550 Bunker Lake Boulevard NW
Andover, MN 55304
(763) 757-3920
anokacountyparks.com

CARVER COUNTY PARKS
11360 US 212 W, Suite 2
Cologne, MN 55322
(952) 466-5250
co.carver.mn.us/parks

CITY OF BLOOMINGTON
1800 West Old Shakopee Road
Bloomington, MN 55431
(952) 563-8877
ci.bloomington.mn.us

CITY OF ST. PAUL
Department of Parks and Recreation
400 City Hall Annex
25 West Fourth Street
St. Paul, MN 55102
(651) 266-6400
stpaul.gov/parks

DAKOTA COUNTY PARKS
14955 Galaxie Avenue
Apple Valley, MN 55124
(952) 891-7000
Trail conditions: (651) 438-4636
www.co.dakota.mn.us/parks

EXPLORE MINNESOTA TOURISM
(888) 868-7476 or
(651) 296-5029
exploreminnesota.com

HENNEPIN COUNTY SERVICE CENTERS
(612) 348-3000

MINNEAPOLIS PARK AND RECREATION BOARD
2117 West River Road
Minneapolis, MN 55411
(612) 230-6400
minneapolisparks.org

MINNESOTA DEPARTMENT OF NATURAL RESOURCES
500 Lafayette Road
St. Paul, MN 55155
(888) 646-6367 or
(651) 296-6157
www.dnr.state.mn.us

MINNESOTA VALLEY NATIONAL WILDLIFE REFUGE
3815 American Boulevard E
Bloomington, MN 55425
(952) 854-5900
fws.gov/midwest/minnesotavalley

MISSISSIPPI NATIONAL RIVER AND RECREATION AREA VISITOR CENTER
120 West Kellogg Boulevard
St. Paul, MN 55102
(651) 293-0200
nps.gov/miss

NATIONAL PARK SERVICE
St. Croix National Scenic Riverway
401 North Hamilton Street
St. Croix Falls, WI 54024
(715) 483-2274 or (715) 483-3284
nps.gov/sacn

RAMSEY COUNTY PARKS AND RECREATION
2015 North Van Dyke Street
Maplewood, MN 55109
(651) 748-2500
co.ramsey.mn.us

THREE RIVERS PARK DISTRICT
3000 Xenium Lane N
Plymouth, MN 55441
(763) 559-9000
Trail hotline: (763) 559-6778
threeriversparks.org

TWIN CITIES METROPOLITAN AREA REGIONAL PARKS SYSTEM MAP AND GUIDE
Metropolitan Council
390 Robert Street N
St. Paul, MN 55101
(651) 602-1000
metrocouncil.org

WASHINGTON COUNTY PARKS DIVISION
11660 Myeron Road N
Stillwater, MN 55082
(651) 430-4300
www.co.washington.mn.us

U.S. FISH & WILDLIFE SERVICE
(800) 344-WILD
fws.gov

IN WISCONSIN
ASSOCIATION OF WISCONSIN TOURISM ATTRACTIONS
100 Wisconsin Avenue, Suite 700
Madison, WI 53703
(608) 250-4873
wiattraction.com

WISCONSIN DEPARTMENT OF TOURISM
201 West Washington Avenue
P.O. Box 8690
Madison, WI 53708
(800) 432-8747 or (800) 372-2737
travelwisconsin.com

WISCONSIN DEPARTMENT OF NATURAL RESOURCES
State Park System
101 South Webster Street
Madison, WI 53707
(888) 936-7463 or
(608) 266-2621
dnr.wi.gov/topic/parks or
wistravel.com

INDEX

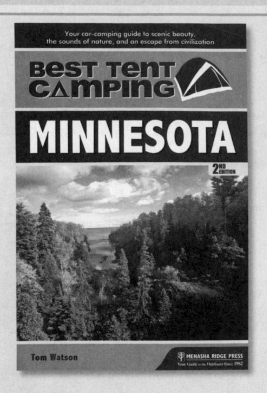
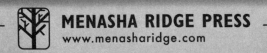

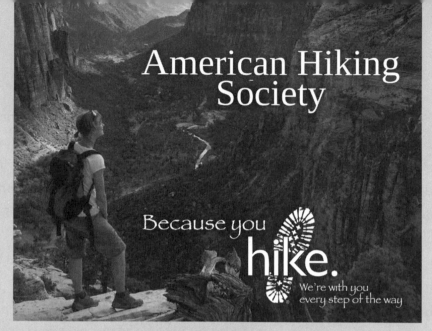

Since its founding in 1976, **American Hiking Society** has been the only national voice for hikers—dedicated to promoting and protecting America's hiking trails, their surrounding natural areas and the hiking experience. **American Hiking Society** works every day:

- Speaking for hikers in the halls of Congress and with federal land managers
- Building and maintaining hiking trails
- Educating and supporting hikers by providing information and resources
- Supporting hiking and trail organizations nationwide

Whether you're a casual hiker or a seasoned backpacker, become a member of **American Hiking Society** and join the national hiking community! You'll not only enjoy great members-only benefits but you will help ensure the hiking trails you love will remain protected and will be waiting for you the next time you lace up your boots and hit the trail.

We invite you to join us today!

American Hiking Society

1422 Fenwick Lane · Silver Spring, MD 20910 · (800) 972-8608
www.AmericanHiking.org · info@AmericanHiking.org

DEAR CUSTOMERS AND FRIENDS,

SUPPORTING YOUR INTEREST IN OUTDOOR ADVENTURE, travel, and an active lifestyle is central to our operations, from the authors we choose to the locations we detail to the way we design our books. Menasha Ridge Press was incorporated in 1982 by a group of veteran outdoorsmen and professional outfitters. For many years now, we've specialized in creating books that benefit the outdoors enthusiast.

Almost immediately, Menasha Ridge Press earned a reputation for revolutionizing outdoors- and travel-guidebook publishing. For such activities as canoeing, kayaking, hiking, backpacking, and mountain biking, we established new standards of quality that transformed the whole genre, resulting in outdoor-recreation guides of great sophistication and solid content. Menasha Ridge continues to be outdoor publishing's greatest innovator.

The folks at Menasha Ridge Press are as at home on a white-water river or mountain trail as they are editing a manuscript. The books we build for you are the best they can be, because we're responding to your needs. Plus, we use and depend on them ourselves.

We look forward to seeing you on the river or the trail. If you'd like to contact us directly, join in at www.trekalong.com or visit us at www.menasharidge.com. We thank you for your interest in our books and the natural world around us all.

SAFE TRAVELS,

Bob Sehlinger

BOB SEHLINGER
PUBLISHER